Please Don't Eat The Wallpaper!

The Teenager's Guide to Avoiding
Trans Fats, Enriched Wheat and
High Fructose Corn Syrup

Dr. Nancy Irven

With Paulette Lash Ritchie

NEW YORK

Please Don't Eat the Wallpaper!

By Dr. Nancy Irven

Compiled, edited and illustrated by Paulette Lash Ritchie

ISBN: 978-1-60037-374-9 Paperback

Library of Congress Control Number: 2007939913

Published by:

MORGAN · JAMES
THE ENTREPRENEURIAL PUBLISHER™

Morgan James Publishing, LLC
1225 Franklin Ave Ste 325
Garden City, NY 11530-1693
Toll Free 800-485-4943
www.MorganJamesPublishing.com

Cover & Interior Design by:

Heather Kirk
www.GraphicsByHeather.com
Heather@GraphicsByHeather.com

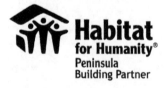

Habitat for Humanity®
Peninsula
Building Partner

ACKNOWLEDGEMENTS

To my patients, who keep teaching me the importance of respecting biochemical individuality.

To my husband, Carl, for his complete support.

To my step-daughter Carla Irven for her expertise in formatting and proofreading.

To Eleanor Lash for her remarkable spelling ability.

To Tom Ritchie for his technological assistance.

DEDICATION

To Judy Powell for inviting me into her classroom to meet and instruct her students.

To the Crystal River High School Health Academy students for sharing their food habits and their trust.

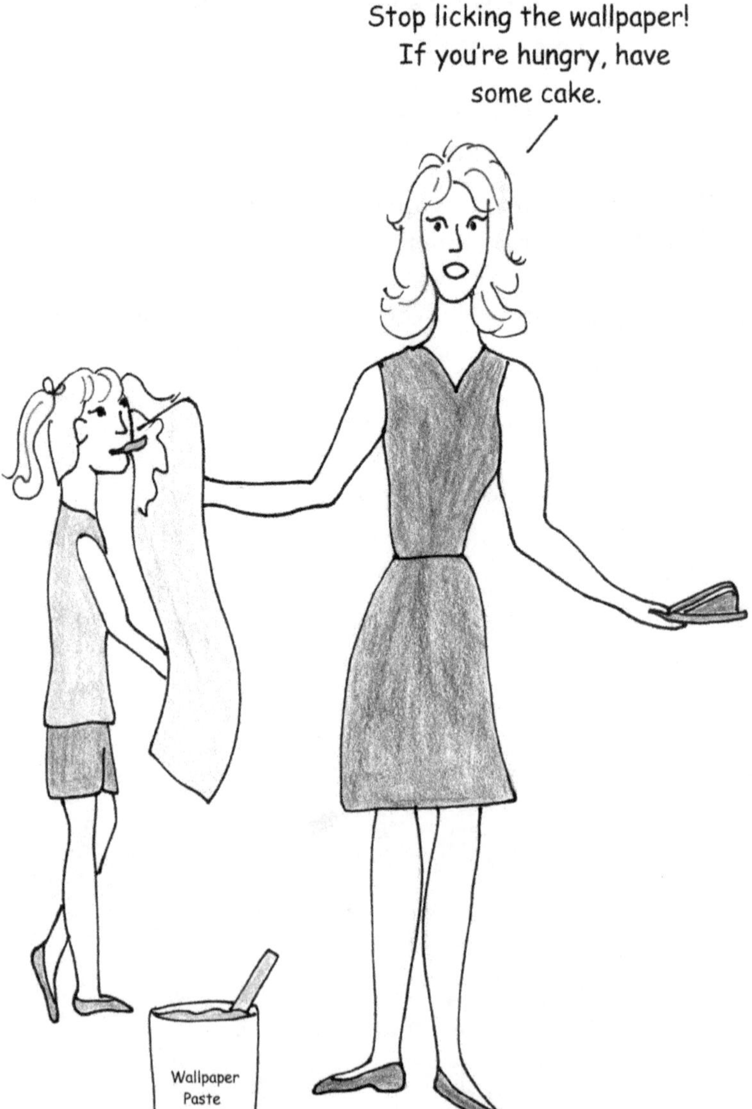
Stop licking the wallpaper! If you're hungry, have some cake.
Wallpaper Paste

INTRODUCTION

When I was a little girl, living on a farm in Kansas, I used to watch my mother cook. She would bake cakes and fry battered chicken and it was all very good. Then one day she decided to redecorate.

I watched her mix the flour with water as if to make a cake, but instead she was making glue to hang wallpaper. I remember thinking, "Didn't she just put that on the chicken last night?"

The realization didn't come until later that when we eat enriched, refined flour in bread, cake, crackers and countless other processed foods, we are eating glue! It took years of research to determine why eating refined and enriched flour is a bad idea. That is part of the reason for this book.

In the course of my studies, I discovered another questionable ingredient in our diets, partially hydrogenated fat, which I will refer to as trans fat. I like to call partially hydrogenated fat, or trans fat, plastic.

I remember my chemistry instructor telling us how the petroleum industry had developed a process to convert petroleum into plastic. He said this new technology had been applied to the food industry to make polyunsaturated oils, which are liquid at room temperature, into margarine, which is solid at room temperature. That was when I understood we now have edible plastic!

These processed oils are called partially hydrogenated fat or trans fat. I strongly stress that partially hydrogenated fat and trans fat are the same thing.

Trans fat (partially hydrogenated fat) essentially has the same chemical makeup as a plastic food storage container! It raises LDL (bad cholesterol) and lowers HDL (good cholesterol), which is the worst possible combination of any fat we can eat. So why do we eat it? We eat it because trans fats are in thousands of products, which give us familiar flavors. These products have been enhanced to be richer in flavor and thicker in consistency.

We have become a society that is addicted to glue (refined flour) and plastic (partially hydrogenated fat). I did a taste test of sunflower seeds with and without trans or partially hydrogenated fat. There was no comparison. The sunflower seeds with the trans fat were much better tasting. I had to make a conscious effort every time I went to the grocery store to choose the sunflower seeds without this form of fat. Now I am satisfied with the better sunflower seed choice. I didn't have to give up a food I enjoyed; I just had to make a better choice.

A third common and harmful ingredient I have found to be prevalent in processed food is high fructose corn syrup. This super sweet substance was introduced into the food supply in the early '70s. Fructose is a naturally occurring sugar found in fruits and some vegetables. High fructose corn syrup is manipulated fructose making it exceptionally sweet. It is bad news for the consumer.

In this book I will explain how these three particular foods affect our health and wellness. I will help the reader determine where they are lurking by examining food labels. And I explain how to avoid them and eat well.

TABLE OF CONTENTS

Introduction VII

Chapter 1 — *The Health Academy Students and Me* 1

Chapter 2 — *What Are Glue, Plastic and Refined Sugar: History and Chemistry* 17

Chapter 3 — *Reading Labels: How Glue, Plastic and Refined Sugars can be Recognized on Labeling of Food Products* 45

Chapter 4 — *Initial Results of the Health Academy Students After Three Years* 61

Chapter 5 — *Food Choices and Meal Planning* 75

Chapter 6 — *Recipes to Get You Started* 85

Chapter 7 — *Excerpts from Letters Written by Students* 91

References 97

Suggested Reading 103

About the Author 105

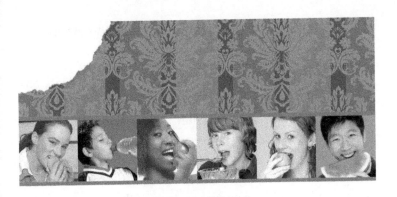

CHAPTER 1

The Health Academy Students and Me

Our local high school contains a health academy for students interested in medical careers. As a board member of the academy, I started a program with the help and cooperation of the academy's director Judy Powell. We were discussing the non-nutritious diets of the students and what we could do about it. We suspected they were not eating healthy foods, but they didn't care.

My first thought was, "do they really know?" I have been providing nutritional consultations in my office since 1995 in which patients provide me with diet diaries for one week. I have reviewed close to 1,000 of these and have discovered that people of all ages are very confused about what is healthy and what is not.

I suggested to Judy that I start a class and teach her academy students what is and what is not healthy and we would see what they would do with the information. We wanted to see if it would make any difference. This began in the fall of 2002. I have taught many classes since then.

I began by measuring the body fat of the students and assigning the writing of food diaries. For three days I asked them to record everything they ate, drank and chewed. Reviewing the diaries I noticed a trend. Most started their days with sugary cereals and low fat, skim or no milk. Lunch was usually an offering of the school system, most commonly pizza and fries with an occasional taco. If they didn't eat what the school served, their lunches were chips and sodas.

Dinners were more varied and it was obvious some of them ate at home. Those dinners were usually a meat, vegetable, bread and dessert. These, as I will explain later, are not necessarily the best foods, but they were better than what the students ate who had fast food dinners. During an entire day there were some students who had nothing but refined sugar.

Here are some examples of actual diaries these students kept in their own words.

EXAMPLE #1

Day one:
Breakfast – None
Lunch – One Coke, pizza, Sprite, whipped cream
Snack – Two bowls of cereal
Dinner – Cream cheese filled poppers, Twizzlers

Day two:
Breakfast – Bowl of almond and vanilla cereal
Lunch – One Coke and some chips
Snack – Coke and a bagel with cream cheese
Dinner – Taco Bell Meximelt

Day three:

Breakfast – Piece of apple, cinnamon muffin, water

EXAMPLE #2

Day one:

Lollypop, herbal tea, submarine sandwich with vegetables, gum, orange juice, gum, apple cider, clump of vitamins, gum, gum

Day two:

Gum, more vitamins, health food bar, gum, Tic-tacs, healthy bar, Sprite, chocolate brownie, rice and mystery contents (school food), gum, Mom's meat stew stuff, gum, health food bar, sherbet, gum

Day three:

Gum, health food bar, gum, vitamins, Oreo, KFC chicken leg, chips, pizza, mystery sandwich, French fries, Sprite, Red Mountain Dew, gum, three gummi bears

EXAMPLE #3

Day one:

Breakfast – Special K cereal bar

Lunch – Pizza, Gatorade

Snack – Popcorn

Dinner – Baked chicken, butternut squash, noodles with alfredo sauce, orange juice

Day two:

Breakfast – Special K cereal bar, orange juice

Lunch – Italian submarine, four Starbursts, two Gatorades, two waters

Dinner – Bowl of chili, water

Day three:

Breakfast – Sausage on English muffin, orange juice

EXAMPLE #4

(This student didn't make it clear what foods were eaten on which day or at which meal.)

Hamburger with lettuce, onions, pickles, catsup and mustard, fries with salt and pepper, Powerade, sip of vanilla milkshake

Macaroni and cheese with pepper, Coke

Pizza, Coke, quepapas

A can of Coke

Two slices pizza, two Poptarts, Sprite, swig of orange soda

Can of Coke

Tacos with meat, lettuce, cheese, sour cream, taco sauce

Two pieces of pizza, orange soda, three glazed doughnuts, milk

Two pieces of pizza and orange soda

Steak and catsup, asparagus with butter and pepper, garlic mashed potatoes, six cookies and milk

3/4 of a bagel and a glass of milk

Gum

Scrambled hamburger and mashed potatoes

Coke (a lot), bagel (untoasted, unsmeared), Honey Nut Cheerios with sugar and milk

EXAMPLE #5

Day one:

1/2 bottle of water

School size chocolate milk

Bowl of salad with two slices of tomato, two cucumber slices, two pieces of ham, spoon of cheese and French dressing

Butterfinger

Saucer of chicken teryaki meal, about 15 pretzels, glass of Coke and Mountain Dew

Day two:

Glass of milk, bowl of grits

Two Tic-Tacs

Bowl of salad with some stuff, bottle of water, can of Coke

Day three:

Glass of milk, waffle with syrup

Five Oreos, can of soda

One small steak, 1/2 bottle water

Gum

EXAMPLE #6

Day one:

Glazed doughnut, water

Pringles, Minute Maid, tea

Spaghetti, Mountain Dew, garlic bread, small chocolate bar

Day two:

Water, Peanut Butter Crunch

Peanut butter and jelly sandwich, Minute Maid, Pringles, Mountain Dew

Water

Fish (two slices), hushpuppy, tea

Day three:

Water, Minute Maid, Sun Chips, chicken, macaroni and cheese, tea, green beans, tea

EXAMPLE #7

Day one:

One piece of gum, one little bag of pretzels, one Powerade

One Powerade, one biscotti, one package of orange peanut butter cookies

One mini bottle of Coke, one little pack of Cheese Nips

Day two:

One piece of gum

One piece of pizza, one Powerade, one Capri Sun

One Nacho Lunchable, one mini bottle of Coke, one can of Coke, one can of Sprite

Six inch Subway sub

Day three:

One hamburger, French fries, one and 1/2 glass Coke

Burrito, chips, one large bowl ice cream with milk

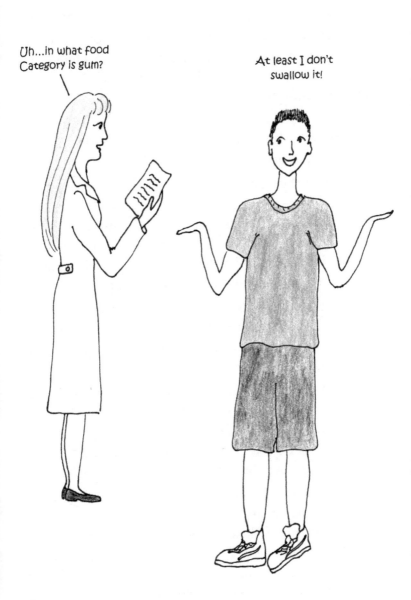

When I analyzed the diets of 24 students over three days I looked at several factors. The data revealed 40% of the students ate no raw food at all. Some examples would be apples, bananas or salads. The students consuming the highest amount of raw foods were the two who ate only four raw foods over three days.

Ninety percent drank soda with an average of four sodas in three days. Three of the teens drank seven sodas in three days. Sixty-eight percent drank no water at all.

In December 2005, Discover magazine published 100 most important discoveries. Number 78 was that Americans are eating as much as 30% non-nutritive food and as a society we have never been as overfed and undernourished. My findings confirmed this with the possibility the numbers could be even worse.

Looking at these diet diaries, I realized the best way for me to explain nutrition to them was to buy the foods they were eating and show them the labels, not just the box that lists the fat and fiber, but the actual ingredients.

When I went to the store to buy them and started examining the labels, I was shocked. The first ingredient was almost always enriched flour. The second or third was often partially hydrogenated fat or high fructose corn syrup. These are probably the three worst items a person can eat.

Armed with what I had bought, I presented foods in two lists: those that are regenerative and those that are degenerative. I did this by dividing the classroom writing board in two, labeling one side regenerative and the other degenerative and we discussed the meaning of the terms. Using Webster's Dictionary, I described regenerative as "to renew by a new growth of tissue." Degenerative means "fallen from a former higher or normal constitution."

I gave them vivid examples of each word. Consider a drooping plant. Water it. The next day it will be tall and perky. Take the same plant and pour gasoline on it. The next day the plant is dead.

The water is regenerative. The gasoline is clearly not good. This example is extreme, but when 30,000 women die yearly from heart-related illness caused by trans fat consumption, I needed to get the students' attention and keep it.

I wanted to be certain they understood this very core concept from Hippocrates: "Let your food be your medicine and your medicine be your food." It was important for the students to understand that food can be a medicine or a poison.

When I hear about food manufacturers debating about whether a food is "bad" for consumers or how "bad" it is, I wonder how the focus got away from good food and good nutrition. If the debate is about how "bad" a food is, then why even eat it at all? Or, as Hippocrates said, it is not medicine.

After we had amply defined the terms regenerative and degenerative, I asked the students to name foods they would put in each category. This is where things got very interesting. This was evidence of how confused people are about food.

The students were quick to raise their hands to tell me with great confidence just which foods were clearly degenerative, or so they thought.

Carbs are bad!

Fats are bad!

Red meat is bad!

Eggs are bad!

Carrots are bad!

Potatoes are bad!

And butter is bad!

Red meat, eggs, carrots and potatoes are all real, whole foods that have been part of human consumption for thousands of years. Yet these students believed they are degenerative. "Carbs are bad" comes from the extremely popular high protein diet. "Fats are bad" comes from the low fat diet phenomenon that has become popular in the past forty years.

The students didn't know what to think. It is no wonder the teens were eating packaged food in which the ingredients are only long chemical names.

After some considerable sorting, we were able to list foods in the appropriate columns. This short list of examples is by no means complete, but I hope it makes my point.

Regenerative foods are such things as vegetables, fruits, meat, eggs, beans, nuts, seeds, whole grains, some fats, dairy foods and some sweeteners (honey, molasses, maple syrup, non-refined sugar). Degenerative foods are enriched/refined grains (glue), partially hydrogenated fat/trans fat/ shortening (plastic), refined-sugars and high fructose corn syrup. A comparison of food lists as it appeared on the board is exampled in Figure 1-1.

FIGURE 1.1

Regenerative Foods	Degenerative Foods
Vegetables	Enriched/refined grains
Fruits	Hydrogenated fats/trans
Meats	fat/shortening
Eggs	Refined sugars
Beans	High fructose corn syrup
Nuts	
Seeds	
Whole grains	
Some fats:	
Butter	
Olive oil	
Coconut oil	
Dairy foods	
Some sweeteners:	
Honey	
Molasses	
Maple syrup	
Non-refined sugar	

I instructed the students to list at least five of their favorite fruits, vegetables, meats, nuts, etc. to encourage them to start adding more of these foods to their diets.

The list of degenerative foods was short, but I decided not to list all the common food chemicals and additives for the students. There are too many. Since enriched/refined grains, partially hydrogenated fat/trans fat/shortening, refined sugars and high fructose corn syrup are very often found to be in the first three ingredients of most packaged foods, I listed them as ingredients to be avoided, thereby automatically trimming a large number of additives and non-nutritive chemicals from the students' diets by association.

For the purposes of this book, however, I would like to list several more refined sweeteners and chemicals that show up on ingredient labels. The long chains of carbohydrate molecules in corn can be broken down and rearranged to make hundreds of different compounds used in food processing or the manufacturing of, well, plastic.

Here is a short list of these: Citric acid, glucose, fructose, high fructose corn syrup, maltodextrin, sorbitol, mannitol, xanthan gum, modified corn starch, unmodified corn starch, dextrins, cyclodextrins, monosodium glutamate, ethanol and lactic acid.

I heard the students say the same things I have been hearing from my patients over the past thirteen years. "You mean I can eat eggs?" "Red meat?" "Potatoes?" "Butter?"

Isn't it amazing that they start their days with breakfast cereals that in most cases contain all the offending ingredients, but they believe eggs are bad for them? I explained to them that for many thousands of years humans have been eating all the foods on the regenerative side of the chart. Only in the past 40 to 100 years have humans been eating glue, plastic and refined sugars as staples in their diets.

Then there is the other piece to the puzzle. In the past several decades the advertising budget for processed foods has been consistently increasing. Last year 10 billion dollars were spent to advertise glue, or refined wheat, plastic, partially hydrogenated fat (trans fat), and non-nutritive sugars to our children, especially on television.

In August 2007, our local newspaper published an article that showed children prefer the taste of milk, carrots and apple juice if they are packaged in McDonald's restaurant packaging, using the familiar golden arches on a red background, even if it was the same product with the packaging removed!

Near the end of class I passed around the packages of food I had found listed in their diaries, which I had purchased. As they read the same ingredients over and over, some of them became angry. I found them saying things like, "I can't believe that this stuff is so bad, but nobody told us."

"Why do our parents let us eat this?"

"Why does the government let us eat this?"

"Why isn't something done about this?"

Then came the inevitable question: "Do you even know what you're talking about Dr. Nancy or are you lying to us?"

Numerous studies have been done in recent years to back up what I have been teaching these students. I will present that information in the next few chapters.

So as not to leave the students in limbo, I also showed them labels of foods that contained no glue, plastic or refined sugars. I wanted to share with them on a more personal level how to eat. I knew I had to feed them.

The following week I borrowed my husband's car and showed up with the back seat and trunk full of food and the utensils needed to prepare it. I wanted to show them how quick and easy it was to wash fresh fruit and vegetables and cut them up.

I prepared a large platter with baby carrots, celery, apple slices and fresh ground peanut butter for dipping. I also provided a platter of cheese and crackers and one of red, yellow and orange peppers, cucumbers, broccoli, and cauliflower with dip. I had quartered oranges, tangerine slices, grapes, almonds, pecans, walnuts, dates, figs and raisins.

I arranged the platters with food combinations so the students could mix the apple slices with peanut butter, the red peppers with dip and the fruit and nuts could be eaten together. I quartered fresh lemon and squeezed it into a glass of water for each of them.

I served toast (using my own toaster brought from home). The students tried two kinds of toasted, buttered sprouted grain breads. They really liked the cinnamon raisin.

We had sandwiches. I used sprouted grain bread to make roast beef, mayonnaise, lettuce, and tomato sandwiches. They also had peanut butter and jelly sandwiches, peanut butter, honey and banana sandwiches and alfalfa sprouts, mayonnaise and tomato sandwiches.

I pulled out my blender and swirled strawberries, blueberries, blackberries, raspberries, bananas and pineapple together with water to create a smoothie that had students coming back for more.

It was quite a food fest and I served absolutely no glue (refined wheat flour), plastic (partially hydrogenated fat) or refined sugar. The students were amazed at how much they enjoyed the foods. Even the diehard glue and plastic addicts who declared they would not have anything to do with it, found some things to their liking.

Judy Powell was eager to share the actions and comments of her students after I left. Many commented on how good they felt the rest of the day. Most were amazed that healthy food could taste so good. She also mentioned noticing some students bringing apples and other fruits, vegetables and nuts to school for snacks and lunches. She also shared with me how the coach commented that several students seemed more focused in practice that afternoon.

The next step was to show the students how to shop. Making arrangements with the manager of a local grocery store, Judy Powell organized a field trip there so I could show the students where I had bought their food. It became apparent that the foods we were seeking could be found around the periphery of the store, in the dairy and meat cases and produce section. Within the aisles as we read labels, we found most of the glue (refined wheat flour), plastic (partially hydrogenated fat) and refined sugar. We found it everywhere.

The store was very generous to the students, providing samples of fresh fruit, vegetables, meats and cheeses. The sample area was set up in the produce section and on several occasions when a student pointed to or inquired about a fruit or vegetable, the store employee would wash it and cut it up for taste testing. The students were impressed.

The final step in my program was to again measure them for body fat at the end of the school semester. Since most of these students were ninth-graders, I followed through by measuring their body fat again before they graduated and interviewed each one.

I will share my findings later. First I will present the facts, studies, history and chemistry of enriched four, partially hydrogenated (trans) fats and high fructose corn syrup.

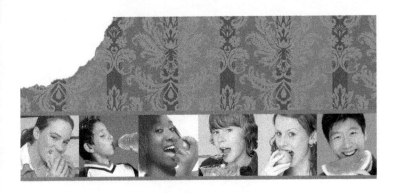

CHAPTER 2
What Are Glue, Plastic and High Fructose Corn Syrup: Chemistry and History

GLUE 》

White bread is appealing. It's soft, mild tasting and, well, nice-looking. White bread seems to be the preferred choice of many people. So what's wrong with that? As we look closer there is actually much wrong with white bread.

Remember, we eat for cell regeneration and good health. Enriched, white flour, which sounds rather healthy (that "enriched" word), has actually been striped of most of the very things we need from grains: fiber, minerals, good fats, protein and antioxidants.

A wheat grain is a kernel with an inedible husk, bran, an endosperm and germ. The nutrients in whole grains are what help protect us from heart disease, stroke, type 2 diabetes, cancer and gastrointestinal ailments. To make enriched flour, the bran and germ are removed from the whole grain, leaving the endosperm. Enriched flour means some nutrients have been returned to the milled flour, but not the germ and bran. Enrichment does add some ingredients to the flour, but the original ones are gone and the returned ingredients are synthetically produced.

Notice in the list of ingredients after the words "enriched flour," the enriched additives are listed as wheat flour, niacin (B), reduced iron, thiamine mononitrate (B1), riboflavin (B2) and folic acid (B9). The synthetic B vitamins are derived from sources you would never consider food. For example, thiamin mononitrate (B1) is synthesized from petroleum. It comes from coal tar from China.

I would prefer my B1 come from the whole grain. The whole grain produced the B1 from the earth's soil, the sun and water. I have a lot of doubt that B1 from petroleum is offering any nutritive value to me. I will go into more detail on synthetic nutrients later.

The germ is the beginning of a new wheat plant. It contains antioxidants, fats, minerals, phytochemicals and vitamins. Phytochemicals are substances found in whole grains, beans, legumes, fruits, nuts and vegetables. They protect the plants from cellular damage that might be caused by their environments. These, in turn, can help protect our cells when we eat them.

There are approximately 99 known phytochemicals in wheat kernels and they are instrumental in disease prevention. They are not retuned to bread flour that has been "enriched." The bran is the edible part of the kernel's husk. It contains the fiber, minerals and phytochemicals.

Why did food manufacturers decide to remove these important food components in the first place? The idea of light-colored bread actually dates back as early as 70 AD. It was preferred by and available to wealthy Greeks and

Romans. It continued to be expensive until the late 1800's when steam engine-powered milling produced white flour that was affordable to the masses.

It was about 1870 in England when the first commercial mills began removing the bran and the germ, about two thirds of the wheat fiber. Thirty years later, still in England, the first documented case if diverticulitis surfaced.

A 2002 Discover Magazine article by Tony Dajer, calls the ailment, "the disease that shows us how we are what we eat." He states that diverticulosis (an out-pouching of the colon) and diverticulitis (an infection of the out-pouching) began to rise rapidly in England after World War I and was directly related to the way flour was milled.

In contrast, he says sub-Saharan Africans who eat a fiber rich diet had absolutely no diverticulitis. Compare that to the city dwellers of Johannesburg who eat refined grains and have common incidences of diverticulitis.

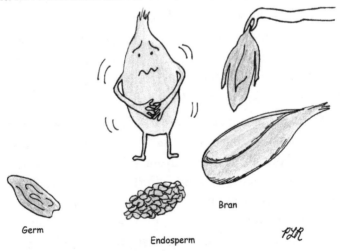

Germ

Endosperm

Bran

PMR

Refining and enriching flour is like stripping the whole-grain wheat kernel naked and handing it a coat to cover up!

A lot of people eat these grains because for decades the food pyramid recommended six to eleven servings of bread, cereal, rice and pasta daily. In fact, this food group was at the very bottom of the pyramid, establishing these foods as staples in our diet.

Whole grain bread, cereal, rice and pasta choices are available but they are not readily found on the shelves of regular grocery stores in the United States. It should be noted that whole grain products while offering benefits can also be detrimental to many people with gluten sensitivity or when consumed in high quantities. It will be further discussed in a later chapter.

One of the biggest problems with enriched flour is the sheer volume of it on grocery store shelves. Take a look the next time you are in a super market or a convenience store. Look at the snacks that line the shelves. Enriched flour will be the first ingredient (which means it is the ingredient in the greatest amount) on most of the labels.

Some health food stores carry a larger selection of whole grain and sprouted grain breads than regular grocery stores, but check labels just the same to make sure you are getting what you think you are getting.

There are also many terms used to mask that a grain is not whole. Manufacturers' use "wheat flour" (of course, it is wheat flour — most flour is made from wheat), "enriched wheat flour," "stone-ground," "fortified, "cracked," "multi-grain," "duram semolina," "unbleached" and "enriched" to make the main ingredient sound better. But as you search the shelves, you will see that even the dark-colored bread appears to be healthy but is not actually whole grain.

In the grocery store bakery where they make the fresh pumpernickel, multigrain and brown breads, if you check the list of ingredients you will first see the word enriched or maybe wheat. If it doesn't say whole wheat, it has been refined. Many of the organic products will say organic wheat. What you are getting is organic glue. Again, if the word "whole" is not there, the whole wheat is not there.

In order for the grain to be nutritionally sound, the very first ingredient must contain the word "whole." That indicates that whole grain wheat is the primary ingredient in the bread. Whole grain may be listed somewhere on the label, but if it is not first, the bread is not nutritionally optimal.

It should be noted that there are some grains we eat that are not milled and do not require the word "whole" to precede them. Examples are wheat berries, millet, corn, popcorn, hulled barley, brown rice, steel-cut oats and associated grains such as quinoa, wild rice and amaranth.

My health academy students thought they were doing well when they listed bread in their diaries, but submarine buns, hamburger buns and enriched bread are close to being empty calories. Unfortunately, there aren't many whole grain bread options in the fast food world. Also unfortunately, those are the restaurants of choice for many teens (and adults). Enriched bread means some nutrients have been returned to the milled flour, but not the germ, bran and phytochemicals.

Unfortunately, fast food restaurants are not the only ones serving refined grains. Almost all restaurants, family, upscale, even those offering fine dining, use enriched grain products for their bread, crackers, pasta and breading.

Unless you can find some trendy "health food" restaurant that advertises whole-wheat pasta and bread, I think I can say with great accuracy that what you are eating is all refined grains. Even that dark-colored loaf some restaurants bring to your table on a cutting board is made of refined grains.

The health risks of refined grains are many. I will cover a few. By removing the bran in wheat and rice, almost all of the magnesium is lost. Magnesium is vital to life. When test animals were deprived of magnesium, they stopped growing and died within 30 days. Magnesium deficiency in humans promotes osteoporosis, cardiovascular disease, hypertension, accelerated atherosclerosis, stroke, anemia, dizzy spells, irritability, low immune function, acne, eczema, psoriasis, senility, impotence, diabetes mellitus, neurological and psychological disorders.

Diabetes is soaring in this country and that has a lot to do with glycemic load, that is, how a food affects blood sugar levels. There is evidence that high glycemic load foods can lead to diabetes by producing high surges in blood sugar.

The Boston Children's Hospital published research through Harvard University's Nutrition Department that revealed two slices of enriched bread had a glycemic load of 4,600 as compared to a can of soda with a glycemic load of 4,100. Two slices of enriched bread have a higher glycemic load than a 12-oz. can of soda! To put this in perspective, a 12 oz. glass of 1% milk has a glycemic load of 900. Researchers in the field of health sciences may use either glycemic load or glycemic index to reveal their findings. Rather than expounding on the differences between them and their relevance, I would like you to focus on the point of the research. An enriched bread sandwich is worse than a soda and together they are a recipe for trouble. Whole grain breads are digested more slowly and have a significantly lower glycemic load.

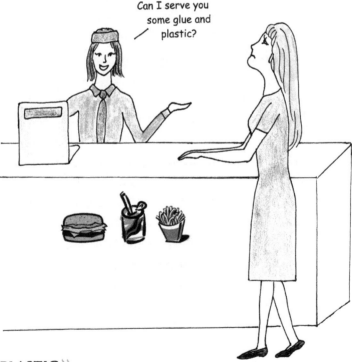

FAST FOOD MENU

Hamburger enrobed in glue.......$1.29
French-fried plastic wrap...........$.98
Concentrated liquid sugar...........$.99

Can I serve you some glue and plastic?

PLASTIC »

Fats can certainly be confusing. There are so-called good fats and bad fats. The body needs fat, but how much is too much? What is trans fat? What is hydrogenated fat?

Let's begin with some definitions.

- **Cholesterol** — This is a common type of body steroid critical in the formation of bile acids, vitamin D, progesterone, estrogens, androgens, mineralocorticoid hormones and glucocorticoid hormones. It is necessary for cell membrane function and is carried in the bloodstream as lipoproteins (fats) and proteins. More than 80 percent of the cholesterol in our body is located inside the cell and makes up the cell membrane. The cell membrane is what allows nutrients into the cell and waste products out.

- **HDL (high-density lipoprotein) cholesterol** — High-density lipoproteins transport cholesterol from the tissues of the body to the liver so it can be excreted. HDL cholesterol is considered good because it is associated with lower heart attack risk.

- **LDL (low-density lipoprotein) cholesterol** — This is often referred to as the bad cholesterol. However it plays a very important role carrying cholesterol to the tissue for deposit. We just don't want too much LDL, because it can indicate the beginning of illness.

- **Saturated fat** — This is a fatty acid (building block of fat) which contains the most hydrogen of the fats. Some sources of saturated fat are butter, lard, coconut oil, palm kernel oil and meat. It is usually solid or almost solid at room temperature.

- **Polyunsaturated fats** — These fats have room for four or more hydrogen atoms and are usually liquid or soft at room temperature. They can be found in safflower, corn, sunflower, and soy oils.

- **Monounsaturated fats** — These fats have room for the addition of two hydrogen atoms and are usually liquid at room temperature. They can be found in olive and peanut oils, as well as avocados and many nuts.

- **Partially hydrogenated fat** — I chose the word plastic to describe partially hydrogenated fats because they utilize the same technology and molecular manipulation as are used in the production of plastic. In simple terms technology can change a long chain hydrocarbon (oil) from a liquid at room temperature to a solid at room temperature, or plastic.

This manipulated fat is called a trans fat or a partially hydrogenated fat. The word trans is used because it means "across from." It refers to the arrangement of the hydrogen atoms and their relation to carbon atoms at the double bond. (Think back to high school chemistry.)

Simply put, liquid corn oil has what is called a cis configuration of hydrogen at the double bond, meaning the hydrogrens are on the same side at the double bond:

$$\begin{array}{ccc} H & & H \\ | & & | \\ C & = & C \end{array}$$

This example is one piece of a chain of similar bonding.

Partially hydrogenated corn oil has a trans configuration of hydrogen at the double bond, meaning the hydrogens are on opposite sides at the double bond:

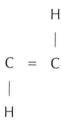

This man-made change in the hydrogen atoms is what we now know is so dangerous to our health. This technology has been applied to the food industry. In 1902, a man-made process of heating vegetable oil to high temperatures and bubbling hydrogen through it in the presence of metal catalysts was used to make vegetable oil, such as corn oil, solid at room temperatures producing shortening. This was very good for food product manufacturers and restaurants. This was very bad for consumers.

When trans fats (partially hydrogenated fats) are used in processed foods, those products have a longer shelf life than when vegetable oil, lard or butter is used. Food that deteriorates or becomes rancid is very expensive to mass-produce.

Partially hydrogenated fat gives foods the thick, rich texture of animal fat and can sit on grocery store shelves for a much longer time. Real fat does not last for more than a few days without decay.

An interesting experiment I share with the students is to put a stick of margarine and a stick of butter in a location where bugs can get to it. Checked on later, the butter will have insect life all over it, feeding off it. The margarine will stay virtually untouched, just as insects would avoid a spill of motor oil on the garage floor.

Now, back to our definitions:

- **Fully hydrogenated fats** — This newest fat has only been on our grocery store shelves for a few years. This is not a trans fat, with hydrogen atoms across the double bonds. This fat has no double bonds. All the carbons are filled with hydrogen.

Fully hydrogenated fat is a man-made saturated fat. If we are going to use saturated fats, why not use the ones nature provides? These include butter, lard and coconut oil. Lard is over 40 percent oleic acid, which is the heart healthy fat in olive oil. I have heard about people who have tried Crisco's new fully hydrogenated shortening. Their opinion was that the piecrusts are not as flaky and the biscuits are a little like rubber. But they concluded at least it wasn't trans fat. They had to give up some taste and texture for health. Oh, well.

Have you ever had pie crust or biscuits made with lard? They are very flaky and tasty. We don't need to give up flavor and texture. We just need to go back to the saturated fats that nature gives us. No one knows what health problems will arise in 20 to 50 years of consuming man-made saturated fat.

Please follow my train of thought for a moment. Trans fats were produced to replace saturated fat, which was supposed to be an unhealthy choice. Now we know that man-made trans fats are the worst fat option. However, conjugated linoleic acid (CLA), a trans fat produced in nature, is actually good for us.

The public is now being sold man-made saturated fat and people believe it is healthier than nature's saturated fats, such as butter. My recommendation is to stay away from the man-made saturated fat completely. To avoid it, read labels.

When you buy lard, the ingredient list will say hydrogenated fat or fully hydrogenated fat. When you buy a product with man-made saturated fat, it will also say saturated fat or fully hydrogenated. You have to look at what oil is used. If the label says fully hydrogenated corn, canola or soy (or any other plant source), then you know it is man-made.

Let me clarify something here. All fats in nature are a combination of saturated and unsaturated fats. Animal fats have more saturated fats. Some tropical seeds, such as coconuts are also higher in saturated fats. Vegetable oils have more unsaturated fats. Even if you eat only vegetables oils, you are still getting some saturated fat. This is the way nature is. Things are blended. There is not just one isolated nutrient or culprit found in any real and whole food.

Saturated fat became known as the "bad fat" which raises cholesterol and contributes to heart disease. That may not be accurate. I will go into more on that later. The fact is trans fat (partially hydrogenated fat) is unquestion- ably dangerous for the heart. Some, such as shortening and margarine, have been proven to lower good cholesterol (HDL) and raise bad cholesterol (LDL). This is the worst possible combination and is causing over 30,000 premature heart disease deaths in women in the United States per year.

That says nothing about American men or men and women in other countries. In fact, research by Harvard Health and Nutrition Department recommends that there is absolutely no safe level of trans fats (partially hydrogenated fats), which means zero in the diet. As far back as 1956, Lancet Medical Journal warned that trans fats were causing heart attacks in large numbers. However in 2006, while this book was in progress, I could not go out to dinner at local or chain restaurants without having my fish and broccoli basted in margarine.

I have asked why some of these places don't even have butter on the premises. I am told it is company policy or they just don't know. Needless to say, I rarely eat out anymore. I'm tired of asking and always getting the same answer. Not knowing what we are eating is very dangerous to our health. Scientific evidence, Ivy League school publications and brief warnings by the media about trans fats (partially hydrogenated fats) do not seem to be trickling down to the awareness of everyday people. So I am going to the schools to tell the students.

I am constantly amazed that, even as the years pass, this is still brand new information for them. In my nutrition practice most of the adults have at least heard that trans fats should be avoided, but they don't know what they are or how to recognize them. This is when I pull out the same box of products I take to the high school, armed with a magnifying glass. The print is so small that even if you know where to look and want to look, you probably won't even be able to see it.

I show them how all of those breads, crackers, cereals, pretzels, cookies, cakes, popcorn, granola bars, kid foods, just about anything in a package contains trans fat (listed as partially hydrogenated fat) in the top three to five ingredients listed. Some of these packages actually advertise zero trans fat, yet when you look in the list of ingredients, there it is! How do they get by with this? By law, if a serving contains less than one half gram it can be advertised as zero.

There has been a huge reduction in serving size to meet this new standard. What chip eater only eats six chips?

I must make it clear, even though it is repetitious, that there is no safe level of trans fat consumption. Most people don't realize that all their shopping for trans fat free products is not working. They appear shocked when I show them it is a staple in their diets. And these are people with the knowledge and motivation to try to keep it out of their diets!

It is also disturbing that we have been told and are still being told that saturated fat, especially in the form of animal products, is contributing to increased levels of cholesterol, increased incidence of heart disease and diabetes. There is so much conflicting and controversial information on this subject. In 1999, a large Harvard study showed that eating eggs every day did not increase a person's chance of having heart disease.

When a person eats a steak, it is roughly fifty percent protein and fifty percent fat. After the steak is grilled, fifty percent of the remaining fat is monounsaturated. Ninety percent of that monounsaturated fat is oleic acid. (Remember the heart healthy fat in olive oil?) That leaves fifty percent of the fat as saturated, but thirty percent of that is stearic acid, which is also healthy.

I have chosen to eat eggs, butter, cream, red meat and coconut oil as staples in my diet. This is not something I recommend to everyone. I respect biochemical individuality. If you prefer vegetable oils instead of animal fats or tropical oils, it is fine by me. My recommendation is to avoid trans fats completely. I have no doubt that any fat found in nature that has been consumed by humans for thousands of years is better than either form of man-made fat.

Please note that animal fats contain a very healthy trans fat (not partially hydrogenated) called conjugated linoleic acid (CLA). This trans fat occurs in higher amounts in animals, which have had adequate physical activity and are grass fed. CLA helps to build lean muscle. In fact, it is so effective that body builders buy it in a synthetic powder form. That, however, would not be my choice. Humans have been consuming CLA in animal tissues for thousands of years. There are not long-term studies on high dose synthetic ingestion of CLA over many years. But, remember what happened with margarine? I am old enough to remember an advertisement about a popular margarine that portrayed a female goddess figure in a garden with the memorable statement, "It's not nice to fool Mother Nature!"

Well, as it turns out, I don't think we can fool nature. I believe our bodies recognize products that are not wholly occurring in nature. It may take years, but the body gets ill when it is not well nourished.

It is my opinion that we not only can't fool nature, we can't replace it when it comes to superior nutrition. I have reviewed countless diet diaries where patients have indicated that it is "bad" to eat beef, butter, egg yolks or cream, but they take powdered CLA. I do not recommend the use of synthetic isolated CLA in large amounts.

Since I deal with teens at the academy, I am very interested in the development of the brains and neurons (nerve cells) of adolescents. These need saturated fat, which contains cholesterol. Some experts are nows recommending at least thirty percent saturated fat in the diet of an adolescent. Eighty percent of the cholesterol in our bodies is in cell membranes, including the cell membranes of the neurons in the brain. That fat is necessary for sustained strength.

Nerves are covered with sheaths made of a substance called myelin. Approximately eight percent of myelin is fat. Nerves carry electrical impulses from the brain to the rest of the body. For an athlete to throw a football or swing a tennis racket, his or her nerves need the necessary fat. Fat is very important in our diets. Studies in Japan are indicating that low cholesterol levels may be associated with strokes and early dementia.

One of my students showed me a diet diary of her previous day: gum, morning vitamins, health food bar, gum, Tic-Tacs, healthy bar, Sprite, chocolate brownie, rice and mystery contents (school food), gum and more gum, mom's meat stew stuff, health food bar, sherbet, gum. She told me one of her teachers looked at it and told her she would be better off without the stew.

When you consider how high in sugar most so-called health food bars are, this student's diet consisted of primarily refined sugars. The only source of fat and protein was her mother's stew, which a respected authority told her, she would have been better off without.

Interestingly, the importance of fat in a youngster's diet is illustrated by how much fat babies need, based on an analysis of human milk. A mother's milk is higher in cholesterol than almost any other food. The fat content is 50%, which is mostly saturated fat and cholesterol. It is essential for the development of the brain. Yet today's market offers low fat baby formula and most of the leading "experts" in nutrition are still giving the same generic advice. Reduce saturated fats to as low as seven percent of the diet. Most of the diets I have reviewed are primarily trans fats (partially hydro-genated fat), refined sugars and refined grains. Most of these patients and students would benefit by adding some animal products, especially animals that are grass fed and have had some exercise or physical activity. For example, wild salmon that swim upstream have higher levels of omega-3 fatty acids than the farm raised salmon.

Just as the nutritional experts are still advising against saturated fat, the advertising budget for milk, featuring a large number of celebrities with milk mustaches, increases. Non-skim, whole milk contains saturated fat. Again, the public is bombarded with conflicting information.

When we eat beef and eggs that are high in CLA and omega-3 fats and fish that are high in omega-3 fats, we are promoting healthy, lean muscle, including the heart muscle. When I see a patient who doesn't want to eat animal prod-ucts I want to understand his or her reason for this choice. There are those who believe they will be healthier without any animal products. However, if a person is abstaining only due to present dietary guidelines and, in fact, would love to eat eggs for breakfast instead of a concoction of refined, synthetic mega dose isolated nutrients and long chemical names packaged in a box or cellophane, I feel compelled to help them feel at ease while eating their eggs.

According to Dorland's medical dictionary, epidemiology is the science concerned with the study of the factors deter-mining and influencing the frequency and distribution of disease. When you begin to study what people eat and what diseases they get, the results are fascinating. Here are some examples taken from Nourishing Traditions by Sally Fallon.

- The Maosai tribe in Kenya and Tanzania eat a diet high in meat, milk and blood — all animal saturated fat. In fact, twice the saturated fat that Americans eat. Heart disease and diabetes are virtually nonexistent. Of course, fruits and vegetables are also included in this diet.

- Native Eskimos eating a primal diet of whale blubber and seals is 80% saturated fat, and they have no heart disease, diabetes, depression, cancer, obesity or hypertension. These diseases only occur if they move into cities and eat refined grains, refined sugars and trans fats (partially hydrogenated fat).

- Yemen Jews living on a traditional diet high in animal fats have no diabetes or heart disease. When they move to Israel, after 25 years in the modern world eating enriched carbohydrates, trans fats (partially hydrogenated fats) and refined sugars, they have incidences of diabetes and heart disease at the same level as everyone else in the cities of Israel.

- Take a look at two cities in India, Udaiper in the north and Madras toward the south, a study of a group of workers who were genetically similar was conducted in both regions. In the north, their diet consisted of ten times the amount of animal fats as were eaten in the south. The people of Udaiper also ate unrefined grains. In Madras, the study group ate refined vegetable oil, such as sesame oil (very low in omega-3 fats), and white rice. Their occurrence of heart disease was 15 times higher than the workers in the north.

● Also, there is the famous French paradox. The French eat a lot of saturated fat in the form of butter, eggs, cheese, cream, liver, meats and pates. The number of middle-aged French men who die of heart attacks each year is less than one half of the number of middle-aged men in the United States who die of heart attacks. In a region called Gascony, where people eat goose and duck liver as a staple of their diets, their rates of heart attack are only one-third that of adults in the United States.

Maybe some of our data in this country is wrong. George V. Mann, Sc.D., M.D., former associate director of the Framingham Heart Study, is quoted as saying, "The diet heart (D/H) hypothesis has been repeatedly shown to be wrong, and yet, for complicated reasons of pride, profit and prejudice, the hypothesis continues to be exploited by scientists, fundraising enterprises, food companies and even governmental agencies. The public is being deceived by the greatest health scam of the century."

William P. Castelli, M.D., director of the Framingham Heart Study stated, "In Framingham, MA, the more saturated fat one ate, the more cholesterol one ate, the more calories one ate, the lower the person's serum cholesterol. We found that the people who ate the most cholesterol, ate the most saturated fat, (and) ate the most calories, weighed the least and were the most physically active."

If you still don't want to eat animal products, then don't. But again, I strongly recommend that you stay away from the trans fats (partially hydrogenated fat).

Not all primal cultures eat such a high percentage of animal meat and dairy. In the hills of Mexico, the Tarahumora Indians have almost no heart disease, diabetes, cancer and other degenerative diseases that plague Americans. They are very physically active, but their diet is high in carbohydrates. A water and ground corn soup is a major component of each meal. They sometimes add pinto beans, squash, mice and/or rabbits, but are often satisfied sipping the corn and water mixture throughout the day.

It isn't necessarily what the healthy people in these cultures are eating that makes the difference. It is what they are not eating — refined grains, trans fats and refined sugars.

REFINED SWEETENERS ⟩⟩

When I took the diet diaries of the students I was teaching and decided to shop for the items, even I was amazed at how often the sweetener high fructose corn syrup was listed on labels. Because of this, I listed it as one of the three ingredients for the students to study and try to remove from their diets. I think high fructose corn syrup (which I will refer to as HFCS) is one of the leading causes of weight problems in this country. The health academy students were eating and drinking gallons of it; in their sodas, fruit juices, cakes, cookies, breads (yes, bread) and even their health food bars.

There are many other names for refined sugars that are most likely just as bad, I didn't want to give the students a long list of don'ts and, since high fructose corn syrup was listed in the first three to five ingredients of almost all the products, I chose it for my classroom presentation.

When I told the students to look for high fructose corn syrup, it wasn't my intention for them to think that if sugar was listed as the first ingredient it was okay. When reading labels, watch for all of these refined sweeteners, which are not regenerative or considered superior nutrition: glucose, fructose, maltodextrins, sorbitol, mannitol, dextrins, and maltose.

This is not to say you can no longer have anything sweet. These sweeteners are not refined and are a better choice when the sweet tooth starts to tingle: raw honey, dehydrated cane sugar juice (succinate), rapadura sugar, molasses, maple syrup, malted barley sugar, brown rice sugar and stevia powder, which is good for diabetics since it doesn't raise blood sugar. There could be more, but I'm attempting to keep this simple.

Refined sugar is detrimental to our health because it is a product that has had the bulk of minerals taken out of it. This causes the body to have to contribute trace minerals for the absorption and assimilation, which means, it takes from the body rather than gives. This is what I call a degenerative food. In 1973 a U.S. Senate committee used the word anti-nutrient to describe processed refined table sugar. The following is a list of the lost nutrients when sugar is refined. I doubt this list is complete: Chromium (93%); Manganese (89%); Cobalt (98%); Copper (83%); Zinc (98%); Magnesium (98%).

This means that when we eat refined sugars our body has to lose precious stores of not easily replaced multiple trace minerals to metabolize the sugar.

I remember reading a couple of stories in William Dufty's book, Sugar Blues. The first one was about a shipwreck in 1793 in which the sailors were carrying a cargo of refined sugar and rum. For nine days they ate sugar and drank rum. When they were rescued they were malnourished and wasted.

The second story was of a young girl who was the sole survivor of a small airplane crash. She subsisted on only snow for 30 days. When she was found, she was not in good shape, but was not considered wasted. The five sailors would not have survived thirty days of refined sugar.

Many studies have been done in which animals on a steady diet of refined sugar died quickly. It is apparent that refined sugar is not just an empty calorie. It is better to eat nothing than to eat refined sugar. In a desperate situation, you could live weeks longer.

When a person is constantly craving sweets, chromium deficiencies have been found as part of the problem. When you look at refined sugar, which has lost 93% of its chromium, you begin to see a cycle. You crave sweets, so you eat chromium deficient sugar, which causes your body to lose some of its stored chromium to metabolize what you have eaten. Your body becomes more chromium deficient and you crave more sugar. This is a cycle of addiction not unlike any drug addiction.

Now that we have established the detrimental effects of refined sugar and its prevalence in processed foods, I would like to move on to high fructose corn syrup. This insidious form of sugar has found its way into thousands of products on grocery store shelves.

It has only been an ingredient in the food supply since the 1970's. The process of producing it involves changing cornstarch into a thick liquid, which is then treated with enzymes, which sweetens it further by producing more fructose. The result is a manmade chemical sweetener made from a natural sweetener and it is significantly sweeter than the unprocessed fructose.

Like trans fat (partially hydrogenated fat), this was another windfall for the food industry. It is a less expensive process than refining cane sugar and food processors can use less of it since it is so super sweet. It also extends shelf life of products containing it. When I switched from a HFCS sweetened jelly to a whole fruit one, I admit my taste buds were very disappointed. I had to train myself to appreciate a sweet that was not so sweet. I've learned to enjoy my jelly now without the "over-the-edge kicker taste."

HFCS is very addictive, in my opinion. It has replaced almost all other refined sugars, because it is so cheap. It also increases profits for the food manufacturers because of the extended shelf life and how it helps prevent crystallization in frozen foods.

Like other refined sugars, HFCS offers no health benefits. There is a possibility it might be even worse. Some studies and publications have reported that HFCS metabolizes differently than other sugars and increases triglyceride levels. My review of diet diaries and blood work shows a correlation between refined sugars and high triglycerides. I cannot isolate HFCS because it is not the only refined sugar that is removed from the diets of my patients. I do see amazing reduction of triglycerides when the refined sugars, including high fructose corn syrup, are removed.

Studies have also shown that high fructose corn syrup does not cause the body to release the hormone leptin, which makes us feel full. This may be true. I have seen people constantly eat foods containing HFCS and they never seem to get full. They can't seem to get enough.

When the hormone leptin is produced it suppresses your appetite after eating. This lets your body know it is full. High fructose corn syrup does not stimulate insulin, which in turn does not trigger an increase in leptin production. Your body has no warning that it is full. When you eat a meal in which the items consumed all have HFCS, you do not get what I call the leptin response. That would be okay every once and a while, but HFCS is very widespread now and the consumer has to look very carefully to avoid it.

So when you have a snack of a soft drink and cookies, in no time, you are back at the refrigerator looking for something else. This is a very serious contributor to obesity. If a person doesn't feel full, he or she is not going to stop eating. It is so easy to eat a lot of foods sweetened with HFCS. In my opinion, HFCS is very addictive.

Because of my work at the high school and teaching students about HFCS, among other ingredients, I have been interviewed and featured in a local newspaper. From there I was interviewed for a piece by a local news station (Fox Channel 13) out of Tampa, Florida. The news program's doctor was presenting a piece on HFCS and was interested in my input. During the course of the interview, I stated that I don't eat any of it in my home and don't eat it at all knowingly. (There are those occasional meals outside the home in which a sauce or a dressing may contain it without my knowledge.) For the most part, I replied that I simply don't eat or drink it.

Within a few weeks I received a package of information from the Corn Growers of America who are the producers of HFCS. The enclosed letter was cordial but assured me of the errors of my views and went to great lengths to educate me with their scientific studies that HFCS is no sweeter and no worse than sucrose — table sugar. My taste buds tell me differently.

But what difference did that make anyway? My point is that all refined sugar has been contributing to diabetes, heart disease, arthritis, osteoporosis, learning disabilities and probably almost every ailment of modern human society.

Is HFCS worse than other refined sugars? Maybe it is or maybe it is not. Time will tell, but if the poison is in the dose, then there is plenty of it in everything. Can we attribute the rise of obesity and diabetes to this one ingredient that showed up in the food supply in the 1970's? I doubt it. Most research is trying to find one reason or ingredient for the deteriorating health in the American population and in cities throughout the world.

In my opinion it is a much bigger problem than just one or a few variables. Even my choice of three — enriched (refined) flour, trans fat (partially hydrogenated fat) and refined sugar, specifically high fructose corn syrup because of its prevalence, is only a part of the big picture. That is why my analysis of the diet diaries looks at many factors.

There are many components to optimal health, but we need to begin somewhere. I think removing the glue, plastic and refined sugars from our diets is a good starting point. Beyond that we could work toward eliminating refined carbohydrates of all kinds and eat meat, vegetables, fruits, whole grains, nuts and seeds that are raised or grown in optimal conditions. We might think about filtering our water and drinking plenty of it. We would benefit by eating more raw foods full of enzymes.

* * * * * *

Before leaving this chapter, I want to make a few comments about the difference between enriched foods vs. whole, intact foods. Foods are made of many components. All foods do not have all components, but we need all of them for optimal health. That is why we need to eat a variety of body friendly foods.

The nutrients we should strive to have in our diets are proteins, fats, carbohydrates, vitamins, minerals, phytonutrients and fiber. Nutrition charts on most food products indicate how much of many of these substances are in the products. But most fall short. It is important to eat whole foods to get all the micronutrients about which we seldom hear.

Whole foods have many, many nutrients. Perhaps I can illustrate this with the analogy between a whole food and a symphony orchestra. In the orchestra there are many instruments blending their sounds into a remarkable harmony. In a whole food there are a huge number of nutrients at work providing excellent nutrition, not just the few we see on a label. A carrot, for example, has over 200 known nutrients and phytonutrients, including dozens and dozens of naturally-occurring compounds of which you probably have never heard: arginine, coumarone, folacin, myristicin, psoralen, suberin, valine, etc.

Some experts estimate that any given whole food has more than 500 synergistic nutrients. When you eat refined foods, such as some grain products, you have reduced a 500-piece professional orchestra to a grade school level five-piece band.

Technology allows food processors to extract chemical structures that look exactly like thiamin mononitrate (B1) or other vitamins from coal tar. When many of these isolated synthetic nutrients are combined for "enrichment" or in a daily multiple vitamin, they are not nutrients in the synergistic harmony of an "orchestra."

Since even the top scientists and researchers still don't know all the nutrients that exist in whole foods — discoveries are still occurring — I am teaching and encouraging patients and students to make whole foods a priority in their diets. Calcium is a common supplement for women. The American Journal of Clinical Nutrition, May 2007 reported that women who get their calcium from food rather than supplements have a higher bone mineral density. They also consume less calcium than those getting it from supplements but they absorb more. Their consumption was an average of 830 mg per day compared to 1033 mg by supplementation.

The research reported that calcium is important to women for estrogen production. Some calcium helps the estrogen production and some calcium doesn't. The calcium from food helps produce estrogen, the calcium from supplementation doesn't. The research also concluded that the type of supplementation determines how much you absorb.

Some calcium, such as calcium carbonate (limestone or oyster shell), does not absorb well. Even our ancestors knew that rocks, oyster shells or coral were not a source of food. A supplemental form of calcium that is much more absorbable is calcium lactate or calcium citrate.

Artificial flavorings, frequently listed as natural flavors, are another example of non-foods that have been heavily introduced into our food supply. Let's compare the artificial vanillin to real vanilla.

Vanillin is widely used to provide that favorite American flavor, vanilla. Even some organic ice cream companies use vanillin instead of real vanilla. What is real vanilla? It is called a bean but is actually the fruit of a rare orchid from Madagascar. The real vanilla extract is rather expensive and somewhere on the label you should see the country, Madagascar, listed.

Vanilla is a very popular flavor and in great demand. Processes abound attempting to make it cheaper and more available. Japanese chemists have recently developed a method to create vanillin from cow dung! Yum!

My point is that our isolated nutrients and "natural" (what's more natural than cow dung?) flavors can come from almost anything. The best way to eat vanilla ice cream would be to make it at home from real cream, eggs, unrefined sugar and vanilla bean extract from Madagascar. With the new ice cream makers on the market, home made ice cream is much easier to make now than when I was a child.

If that is still too much work, on a hot summer's day if I want something to eat that is cold, sweet and wet, I reach for any of the varieties of melon. Watermelon is one of my favorites.

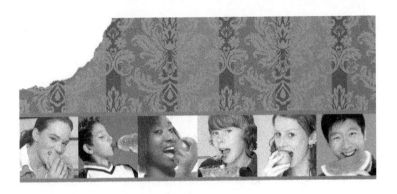

CHAPTER 3

Reading Labels: How Glue, Plastic and Refined Sugars can be Recognized on Labeling of Food Products

Deciphering labels does not require a degree in advanced food science. There is a lot of information in the nutrition facts listed on food packages and it can be important to individuals with any number of concerns.

Diabetics need to look for carbohydrates and sugars. Dieters might be interested in serving size and the calorie count. For the purposes of this book, though, the label should be consulted to find trans fat (partially hydrogenated fat), enriched flour and high fructose corn syrup. It used to be a lot more difficult to determine the amount of trans fat in a product, but thanks to legislation that took effect in January 2006, trans fats must now be listed in nutrition facts. Check for that first.

The best place to look for specific components of a particular product is the ingredient list at the bottom of nutrition facts. If enriched flour is the first item in the list of ingredients on say, bread or crackers, that product should be avoided. Instead look for "whole" in the description of the wheat. "Made with whole wheat" is one way manufacturers try to sway consumers into thinking their product is healthy. If whole wheat isn't the first ingredient, keep looking for another brand.

There are several breads that do pass that criteria, but fail further down the list. An astonishing number of breads also list high fructose corn syrup as an ingredient. Why do we need high fructose corn syrup in bread? Keep looking. There are breads made without trans fat, enriched flour and high fructose corn syrup. They are few, but they do exist.

Remember, a product can say it has zero trans fat, but still have small amounts of it. Be sure to check for partially hydrogenated fat in the ingredient list. I recommend avoiding that product completely. Again, there is no safe level of trans or partially hydrogenated fat!

When I took the high school students to the grocery store, it was to help them identify the products that contained plastic, glue and refined sugar. They were amazed at the difficulty of finding products without those ingredients. They found the good food in the produce section, fresh meats, much of dairy, and the aisles containing raw nuts, beans and whole grains.

A rule of thumb is to avoid processed foods as much as possible. Many grocery stores that have health food sections (isn't it interesting that food can actually be separated into healthy and unhealthy?) offer a good place to look for whole grain products. Some health food stores have a larger selection of whole grain and sprouted grain products, such as pita bread, English muffins, tortilla shells, hamburger buns, submarine sandwich buns and pasta, but good food can be found in regular grocery stores.

Here are examples of popular products I have chosen because I see them as staples in a majority of the diet dairies I review. I have reviewed the lists of ingredients and have categorized the foods as nutrient deficient, better choices and excellent choices. Copyright laws have limited me so I will not reveal the names of any of these products. The following reproduction of a nutrition facts label gives you an idea of what to look for when shopping.

Nutrition Facts

Serving Size 16 Crackers (30g)
Servings Per Container   About 9

Amount Per Serving

Calories 140 Calories from fat 45

	% Daily Value *
Total Fat 5g	**8%**
Saturated Fat 1g	**5%**
Trans Fat 1.5 g	
Cholesterol 0 mg	**0%**
Sodium 290 mg	**12%**
Total Carbohydrate 21g	**7%**
Dietary Fiber 1g	**6%**
Sugars 3g	
Protein 3g	

Vitamin A   0% ● Vitamin C 0%

Calcium   0% ● Iron   6%

*Percent Daily Values are based on a 2,000 calorie diet. You daily values may be higher or lower depending on your caloric needs:

	Calories	2,000	2,500
Total Fat	Less than	65g	80g
Sat. Fat	Less than	20g	25g
Cholesterol	Less than	300mg	300mg
Sodium	Less than	2,400mg	2,400mg
Total Carbohydrate		300g	375g
Dietary Fiber		25g	30g

Calories per gram:
Fat 9 ● Carbohydrate 4 ● Protein 4

INGREDIENTS ENRICHED FLOUR (WHEAT FLOUR, NIACIN, REDUCED IRON, THIAMIN MONONITRATE [VITAMIN B$_1$], RIBOFLAVIN [VITAMIN B$_2$], FOLIC ACID), PARTIALLY HYDROGENATED SOYBEAN AND/OR COTTONSEED OIL WITH the FOR FRESHNESS, WHOLE GRAIN WHEAT, SUGAR, DEFATTED WHEAT GERM, WHOLE GRAIN OATS, SALT, CONTAINS TWO PERCENT OR LESS OF HIGH FRUCTOSE CORN SYRUP, MALTED BARLEY FLOUR, ARTIFICIAL COLOR (ANNATTO AND TURMERIC EXTRACTS), SOY LECITHIN.

Here are some things to look for when examining a food label:

Trans fat – Don't buy it if there is trans fat in the ingredients.

Watch for three main things in the ingredients. You want to avoid enriched flour as the first or second ingredient. That means empty calories.

Partially hydrogenated fat and high fructose corn syrup are also ingredients to be avoided.

When you look at a label, immediately check for trans fat. If there is trans fat in the product, I strongly suggest you put it back. If the amount of trans fat is listed as zero grams, remain suspicious.

Go to the list of ingredients. You will see that many products list glue, plastic and refined sugars as the first three to five ingredients. The ingredients are listed in order of quantity. The ingredient with the highest quantity is listed first. The second has the next highest amount and so on.

When I go over labels one-on-one with patients, I have learned their first concern has been to look at the top of the table for grams of fat or grams of carbohydrates. They seem to have been programmed to think in terms of one or the other of two very popular current diet choices: low fat or low carbohydrate. If you don't look at the source of the fat or carbohydrate, you are probably only comparing grams of glue and plastic to grams of glue and plastic.

The bottom of the label where you see the word "INGREDIENTS" is the where you will find the most important information on the package. Remember, we want our carbohydrates, fats, proteins and fiber to come from real, whole nutrient-dense food. Make every calorie count toward superior nutrition!

Now let's look at labels.

The following are lists of packaged foods. I begin with what I consider very nutrient deficient foods. Later I list better choices and some excellent choices.

BREADS 》

Nutrient deficient

My first example is a list of actual ingredients from a popular white bread marketed to children. "Ingredients: Enriched wheat flour [flour, barley malt, ferrous sulfate (iron), "B" vitamins (niacin, thiamine mononitrate (B1), riboflavin (B2), folic acid)], water, high fructose corn syrup, soy and/or cottonseed fiber, yeast, wheat gluten, calcium sulfate. Contains 2 percent or less of: soybean oil, salt, dough conditioners (may contain: sodium stearoyl lactylate, mono and diglycerides, calcium dioxide, dicalcium phosphate, sorbic acid and/or datem), soy flour, yeast nutrients (may contain: ammonium chloride, ammonium phosphate, ammonium sulfate and/or monocalcium phosphate), vinegar, cornstarch, wheat starch, enrichment [Vitamin E acetate, ferrous sulfate (iron), zinc oxide, calcium sulfate, niacin, Vitamin D, pyridoxine hydrochloride (B6), folic acid, thiamine mononitrate (B1) and Vitamin B12], enzymes, whey, calcium propionate (to retain freshness), soy lecithin."

This bread is marketed to children and yet the first ingredient is still enriched flour (glue) and it contains high fructose corn syrup. Keep in mind, the isolated synthetic vitamins, such as thiamin mononitrate (B1), are processed from petroleum, which is coal tar from China. Also, the numerous chemicals listed do not indicate superior nutrition.

Better Choice

A better choice for bread is whole wheat bread. This bread does have refined sugar, which is why I don't list it as an excellent choice. "Ingredients: 100% stone ground whole wheat flour (malted barley flour), water, sugar, non-fat dry milk, soybean oil, salt, honey, yeast, wheat gluten, malt, calcium propionate added to retard spoilage."

Excellent Choice

Bread made of sprouted grains is a nutrient dense, excellent choice. "Ingredients: organic sprouted wheat, organic sprouted barley, organic sprouted millet, organic malted barley, organic sprouted lentils, organic sprouted soybeans, organic sprouted spelt, filtered water, fresh yeast, sea salt."

The sprouted grain bread uses sprouted organic grains. It is sweetened with organic malted barley, which is a whole, unrefined food. The interesting thing about this bread, is that when you take a grain and allow it to sprout before you turn it into bread, it no longer contains the protein gluten, which is found primarily in barley, rye and wheat, whole and enriched.

Estimates in this country are that one in 130 people have a "gluten sensitivity," which can cause digestive problems. By eating this bread, you are not only getting superior nutrition, you are eliminating a possible "unknown factor" in the digestive problems many people experience. There are plenty of sprouted grain breads on the market in a wonderful variety of loaves, English muffins, tortilla shells, hamburger buns, sub sandwich rolls, pita bread and even breakfast cereals.

When I teach about the three main ingredients to avoid, I don't mean to imply that a product that does not contain them (refined grain, partially hydrogenated fat and refined sugar) is necessarily considered superior nutrition. For example, one seemingly healthy bread lists the following ingredients: "Stone ground whole wheat flour, water, mali-tol, wheat gluten, yeast, contains 2% or less of each of the following: butter, salt, dough conditioners (sodium steroyl lactylate, calcium stearoyl-2-lactylate, monoglycerides, calcium iodate, ethoxylated mono and diglycerides, calcium peroxide), cultured whey, vinegar, natural flavors, calcium sulfate, monocalcium phosphate, yeast food (ammonium sulfate)."

As you can see, the grain is whole. There is no partially hydrogenated fat and no high fructose corn syrup. However, it does contain a lengthy list of isolated nutrients and chemicals. When you compare this list to the sprouted grain bread, you can see a big difference between long chemical names in one and recognizable foods in the other. Avoiding the three primary ingredients is only the beginning, but I chose them because of their prevalence.

Let's move on to crackers. Here are two examples of popular crackers used in many restaurants.

CRACKERS 》

Nutrient deficient

"Ingredients: Enriched flour (wheat flour, niacin, reduced iron, thiamin mononitrate (vitamin B1), riboflavin (vitamin B2), folic acid), partially hydrogenated soybean and/or cottonseed oil with TBHQ for freshness, sugar, contains 2% or less of salt, leavening (baking soda, sodium acid pyrophosphate, monocalcium phosphate), high fructose corn syrup, corn syrup, sodium sulfite, soy lecithin."

"Ingredients: Enriched Flour (wheat flour, niacin, reduced iron, thiamine mononitrate (vitamin B1), riboflavin (vitamin B2), folic acid), soybean oil, salt, partially hydrogenated cottonseed oil, baking soda, malted barley flour, calcium carbonate (source of calcium) yeast."

Notice the first popular cracker has all three of the offending ingredients. Enriched flour (glue), partially hydrogenated soybean and/or cottonseed oil (plastic) and high fructose corn syrup, as well as, two other refined sugars listed as "sugar" and "corn syrup."

The second popular cracker's first ingredient is again the enriched flour (glue) and it contains partially hydrogenated cottonseed oil (plastic). These are the soda crackers I was given as a child when I was sick with the flu. Many of my patients who have been educated about reading labels have told me that when they got sick, they automatically bought these crackers without even reading the label. We do trust our upbringing and when we are sick we tend to reach for those "comfort foods" we were given as children. However, glue and plastic are not what a sick body needs.

A homemade chicken and vegetable broth would offer thousands of healing nutrients in the perfect synergistic amounts to nourish a sick body. Remember the 200 ingredients in the carrot? Now add some onions, celery, garlic and chicken. The nutrients are innumerable and could not even begin to be listed on an ingredient label.

Better Choice

"Ingredients: Whole rye, corn bran, salt, and caraway."

Now, about the better choice: there are several crackers that have similar ingredients and they are generally located in grocery stores' bread aisles. The rest of the crackers with refined sugars and partially hydrogenated fats are located in the cookie aisle.

If you compare the ingredients of the crackers found in the cookie aisle with the cookies, the similarities are astonishing. People eat crackers as a snack because they think they are healthier than cookies. This is not always so. Many people, given a choice between the cookie and the cracker and told they are both equally healthy, would choose the cookie. I'm explaining this because there are some complaints that the seemingly better choice crackers don't taste very good.

In my opinion, a cracker is like rice or pasta. It tastes like what you put on it, such as cheese, tuna salad or peanut butter. If you want to eat a cracker that tastes sweet and buttery all by itself, what you really want is a cookie. Well then, have the cookie! We should stop fooling ourselves that those tasty crackers in the cookie aisle are better for us than the cookies.

What are more heavily marketed and more popular with children and many adults for starting the day, than cereals? Let's take a look.

BREAKFAST CEREALS 》

Nutrient deficient

This is an example of a colorful cereal marketed toward children. "Ingredients: Sugar; corn flour; wheat flour; oat flour; partially hydrogenated vegetable oil (one or more of coconut, cottonseed, and soybean); salt; sodium ascorbate and ascorbic acid (vitamin C); niacinamide; reduced iron; natural orange, lemon, cherry, raspberry, blueberry, lime and other natural flavors; red #40; blue #2; zinc oxide; yellow #6; turmeric color; pyridoxine hydrochloride (Vitamin B6); blue #1; riboflavin (Vitamin B2); thiamin hydrochloride (Vitamin

B1); annatto color; Vitamin A palmitate; BHT (preservative); folic acid; Vitamin B12; Vitamin D."

The first ingredient in the children's cereal is refined sugar. It contains refined wheat flour (glue) and partially hydrogenated vegetable oil (plastic). It also contains several artificial coloring agents. These are not the raw materials for a healthy brain. I would not start my day with this and would not recommend it for children.

Better Choice

"Ingredients: Whole Oat Flour, Un-sulphured Molasses, Whole Wheat Flour, Ground Almonds, Wheat Germ, Baking Soda, Sea Salt, Natural Flavor, Vitamin C, Natural Vitamin E."

Excellent Choice

Homemade Oatmeal — Ingredients: steel cut oats cooked with raisins, nuts and fruit (such as apples) flavored with cinnamon and nutmeg and sweetened with real, non-processed maple syrup or molasses.

I get numerous questions from students and patients concerning breakfast cereals. I have chosen not to eat boxed cold cereals. I have not eaten them for many years. A few years ago when the "healthy" food market began to provide organic grain boxed cold cereals to our local grocery store, I decided to try one.

Since I hadn't eaten any cold cereals for so many years my taste buds may have been less dulled. I immediately tasted that old familiar flavor of a fried grain, as in a chip. Only this time I didn't taste salt, I tasted sugar! I concluded that boxed cold cereals are sugar-flavored fried grains.

Through my studies I have learned a little something about how cereal is made. The method involves pushing a cereal "grain paste" through an extruder at a high temperature, which produces each little different shape (a circle, square, etc.) of the cereal. This paste has been heated to 200°F or more, which gives it the "fried" flavor.

I counted the variety of cereals in the grocery store. There were over 300! Sixty-five were in the health food section and 250 in the regular section. Cold breakfast cereals have not been part of human consumption for thousands of years. When my grandmother went to the grocery store in the early 1900's, she did not have a choice of over three hundred boxed cold cereals. She ate eggs, meat, fruit, whole grain hot cereals and breads for breakfast. She ate the same way people all over the world have eaten for thousands of years.

When I look at the ingredient list of a bag of potato chips: "potatoes, safflower oil and salt" or corn chips: "whole corn, corn oil and salt," I wonder if I could convince parents that their children could be better off starting their day with a respectable chip? Most people could never accept that a chip may have less offending ingredients than a breakfast cereal because of the way breakfast cereals are marketed. But neither is superior nutrition, especially for the developing brain of a child starting the day. However, on occasion I do enjoy a respectable corn chip with a great salsa.

Now that I have mentioned chips, which are usually snacks, not breakfast, consider the ingredient label on a popular pretzel. Many patients and students choose pretzels for snacks because they consider them a healthy option.

SNACKS >>

Nutrient deficient

Now here's that pretzel. "Ingredients: Enriched wheat flour (contains niacin, reduced iron, thiamine mononitrate, riboflavin, and folic acid), salt, corn syrup, partially hydrogenated soybean oil, yeast, sodium bicarbonate."

Notice the enriched wheat (glue), partially hydrogenated soybean oil (plastic) and corn syrup. If you are craving a salty and crunchy snack you can choose nuts and popcorn. Remember to read labels.

Here's another seemingly harmless snack. This one can be found in non-acceptable and acceptable forms. Look at one of the very popular microwave popcorn products. "Ingredients: Popcorn, salt, partially hydrogenated soybean oil, high monounsaturated canola oil, artificial and natural butter flavors, color added."

Notice the partially hydrogenated soybean oil (plastic). Popcorn may be healthy but edible plastic is not!

Excellent Choice

Popcorn kernels popped at home with a hot air popper or a heavy saucepan on the stove with some butter added.

Nuts are another very healthy snack. However, avoid products with labels like these:

"Ingredients: Peanuts, sugar, honey, corn syrup, peanut and or cottonseed oil, salt, fructose, cornstarch, xanthan gum."

"Ingredients: Cashews, salt, cornstarch, sugar, monosodium glutamate (flavor enhancer), maltodextrin, gelatin, corn syrup solids, dried yeast, paprika, onion and garlic powders, spices, natural flavors."

Instead try ingredients containing only pecans, walnuts, almonds or roasted peanuts in their shell with or without salt.

Peanut butter is a staple on the diet diaries of many of the students. Peanut butter is a very good source of healthy fats and proteins but, as with many other foods, check the labels.

PEANUT BUTTER ⟩⟩

Nutrient deficient

This first listing is a very popular peanut butter. "Ingredients: roasted peanuts and sugar; contains 2 % or less of molasses, partially hydrogenated vegetable oil (soybean), fully hydrogenated vegetable oils (rapeseed and soybean), mono and diglycerides and salt."

Notice the refined sugars, partially hydrogenated fat, and fully hydrogenated vegetable oils that are in the popular brand.

Better Choice

"Ingredients: Peanuts and salt."

Excellent Choice

"Ingredients: Fresh ground peanuts."

SANDWICH SPREADS ⟩⟩

When I made sandwiches for the students I used mayonnaise. I get a lot of questions about that. In my opinion, the ingredients, even though they contain a small amount of refined sugar, are better than the popular mayonnaise replacement, salad dressing. Look at the difference in the labels:

Nutrient Deficient

Mayonnaise substitute or salad dressing is a commonly used condiment. "Ingredients: Soybean oil, water, vinegar, high fructose corn syrup, eggs, sugar, modified food starch, starch, salt, mustard flour, spice, paprika, potassium sorbate as a preservative, natural flavor." Notice the high fructose corn syrup and sugar in the mayonnaise substitute. Some of these products advertise they are low in fat. I find most products that have removed the fat, have also added sugar.

Better Choice

Mayonnaise is a better choice. "Ingredients: Soybean oil, water, eggs, vinegar, contains less than 2% of egg yolks, lemon juice concentrate, salt, sugar, dried onions, dried garlic, paprika, natural flavor, calcium disodium EDTA as a preservative."

Excellent Choice

Homemade mayonnaise: eggs, salt, vinegar or lemon juice, unrefined sugar, dried mustard, cold-pressed salad oil, (i.e. safflower, sunflower or corn).

This is the same with BBQ sauces, salad dressings and an array of condiments that are used as staples in our diets. When trying to avoid fat in the form of healthy oils, cream, eggs, butter, etc.; we end up with products that are full of long chemical names and much higher in sugar.

Speaking of sandwich spreads and butter, I would like to mention margarine and other margarine-like products.

They have been heavily advertised as heart healthy, but, again, read the labels.

BUTTER AND MARGARINE ⟩⟩

Nutrient deficient

This is the ingredient list of a well-known margarine: "Liquid soybean oil, partially hydrogenated soybean oil, water, whey, salt, vegetable mono- and diglycerides and soy lecithin (emulsifiers), potassium sorbate and sodium benzoate (to preserve freshness), artificial flavor, phosphoric acid (acidulant), Vitamin A palmitate, colored with beta carotene (source of Vitamin A). Contains: Milk, soy."

Here is another margarine. This one advertises on its label that it has zero trans fat. "Ingredients: water, plant sterol esters, liquid soybean oil, liquid canola oil, partially hydrogenated soybean oil, salt, whey (milk), vegetable mono- and diglycerides, (potassium sorbate, calcium disodium EDTA) to protect quality, soy lecithin, polyglycerol esters, lactic acid, Vitamin E, artificial flavor, beta carotene (color), Vitamin A (palmitate)."

Notice the partially hydrogenated fats in both of these yellow-colored food imposters.

Better Choice

Butter: "Ingredients: Sweet cream, salt."

* * * * * *

I cannot list thousands or even hundreds of labels in this book. I can teach you how to read them and encourage you to do so. Until you establish your staples, (i.e. a favorite bread, cracker, salad dressing, sandwich spread, etc.) please read every label of every product you pick up to use or buy. After a while you won't have to re-read the same label, since you will have decided it is healthy enough for you and your family. You will be able to grocery shop quickly as the majority of your foods will come from produce (very few labels there), meat, dairy, beans, whole grains and nuts.

Remember, any product that has not been consumed by humans for thousands of years is probably refined or man-made. It is very likely not a source of superior nutrition. It should not be consumed daily as a staple. Foods without labels are usually healthier. Think of fruits and vegetables. On most ingredient labels, the healthier foods have a shorter list of ingredients.

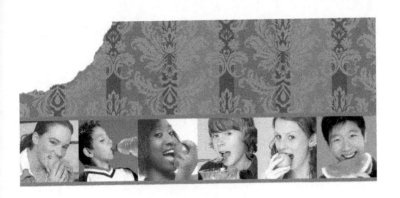

CHAPTER 4
*Initial Results of the Health Academy
Students After Three Years*

After three years the students were asked to have their body fat measured and to participate in an oral exit interview. I asked four primary questions: Do you remember the three ingredients about which you were taught in my class? Have you been reading labels to identify these ingredients? Have you made any dietary changes as a result of learning this information? Has there been any change in your level of physical activity?

The answers were varied. Some remembered all the ingredients, were reading labels and making significant changes in their diets. Some students remembered one or two of the ingredients, had not been reading labels, but had still made some dietary changes. Some students didn't remember anything and had made no dietary changes or changes in physical activity.

Most of the students could list a few dietary changes and I was pleased that one of the most frequent changes was the reduction or cessation of soda drinking and the addition of more water. In my opinion that was a very important modification, even if it was the only one those students made.

After the body fat measurements, I saw that many of the students had a decrease in visceral body fat. Almost all the students who showed a decrease were those who participated in sports or some type of physical activity. Interestingly, earlier, when I had done body fat measurement after only three or four months, I saw that students who were active showed the quickest reduction.

The students who made dietary changes to remove the detrimental ingredients and replace them with fresh food without physical activity did not show significant body fat loss in only three or four months. Optimal health cannot exclude exercise and physical activity. However, a study of professional athletes shows that physical activity alone does not exempt them from cardiovascular disease, diabetes, osteoporosis and all the rest of the degenerative diseases that are so rare among the people who eat more primal diets. Plus the people who live in cultures with primal diets tend to be more active. It is just their way of life.

Overall, I am impressed with most of the results of this study. I would like to share one case in which the student made no dietary changes and got no regular physical activity.

This is her initial diet diary written in February 2003.

Day one:
Breakfast – Life cereal
Snack – pretzels
Drink – lemonade

Lunch – some (not a whole bag) sour cream and onion chips, four crackers, half a honey bun, one bite of an ice cream sandwich, blue Gatorade

Snack – five or six cheese puffs

Dinner – three pieces of turkey bacon, one fried egg, hash browns, grapefruit juice

Day two:

Breakfast – Life cereal

Snack – two chocolate chip cookies

Lunch – pizza, one eighth of a honey bun

Dinner – chicken, broccoli, bread, milk

Day three:

Breakfast – Life cereal

Snack – sour cream and onion chips

Lunch – pizza, one quarter honey bun, ice cream sandwich

Dinner – Spaghetti, milk

Day four:

Breakfast – Coke

These were her February 2003 statistics:

Height: 56"

Weight: 78 lbs.

Body Fat: 28% (Optimal visceral body fat for her age is 15-26%)

Body Mass Index: 16 (This is a calculated relationship between height and weight. In this example, the student was visibly thin and appeared underweight.)

Her follow-up statistics:
Height: 56 1/2"
Weight: 87 lbs.
Body Fat: 35.4%
Body Mass Index: 17

She had an increase of over 7% visceral body fat in two and a half years of high school. At her exit interview, she stated she had made no dietary changes since her initial diet diary and she was not getting any regular physical activity. At 87 pounds, she has a visual appearance of being very thin and possibly underweight. However, the consistency of her tissue was very high in fat.

I used a Futrex 5000A to measure the body fat in the study. Unlike the induction current used in many home scales and inexpensive measuring devices that don't measure visceral fat, the Futrex 5000A uses near infrared to measure visceral fat. The cost of the machine was approximately $4,000. The accuracy of the Futrex 5000A is comparable to the use of magnetic resonance imaging (MRI) and computed tomography (CT). MRIs and CTs are very expensive in dollars and time. I have mentored science projects since 2001 for the local high school health fair and we were able to assess the visceral fat of over 120 students during a five-hour period each year.

Visceral fat does not show outwardly in an obvious way. It wedges itself between muscle fibers as a marbling of fat within the muscle tissue. It also wedges between and around the organs.

According to the Harvard Woman's Health Watch, this type of fat distribution can increase the risk for cardiovascular disease, Type 2 Diabetes and is linked to breast cancer and gallbladder disorder.

What causes this fat? A very simple answer would be to look at how marbling is achieved in a tender, juicy steak, which costs more because of the extra fat it contains. The animal is fed in a pen (no exercise) and fed grains (high carbohydrate diet). You won't see this fatty tissue in any wild animal. Grass fed animals that get a lot of exercise, have leaner tissue and higher levels of CLA, the healthy trans fat.

According to a prominent cardiologist, Dr. Roger Blumenthal at John Hopkins Hospital, the visceral fat acts like the fuel depot for cholesterol. It is fed into the liver and releases the artery-choking LDL cholesterol. "It's the fat you don't see that kills you," Dr. Blumenthal warns.

The same Harvard Woman's Health Watch previously mentioned adds that scientists are discovering visceral fat produces more chemicals from the immune system, which produce low levels of inflammation, insulin resistance and cardiovascular disease. Many of the chemicals have not even been identified, but they may be contributing to blood clotting and high blood pressure

Lack of physical activity and too many nutrient deficient carbohydrates are two primary factors contributing to this pandemic of fatty tissue in the human population. Obesity statistics are based on a body mass index of 30 or over. Figure 4.1, on the following page, is a typical chart on Body Mass Index also referred to as BMI. Body Mass Index is a relationship between your height and weight. To use the chart, locate your height in the left column, then move across the row to locate your weight. The number at the top of the column is your BMI. A BMI of 19 to 26 is healthy, 27 to 29 is considered overweight and 30 and over is obese. However, my experience measuring visceral fat since 1999 in my patients and 2001 in the high school students (almost 2,000 measurements so far) reveals that many people who are visibly slender are carrying excessive and dangerous levels of visceral fat.

FIGURE 4.1

BODY WEIGHTS IN POUNDS ACCORDING TO HEIGHT AND BODY MASS INDEX													
	Body Mass Index (kg/m2)												
	19	20	21	22	23	24	25	26	27	28	29	30	35	40
Height	Body Weight (lb.)												
4'10"	91	96	100	105	110	115	119	124	129	134	138	143	167	191
4'11"	94	99	104	109	114	119	124	128	133	138	143	148	173	198
5'0"	97	102	107	112	118	123	128	133	138	143	148	153	179	204
5'1"	100	106	111	116	122	127	132	137	143	148	153	158	185	211
5'2"	104	109	115	120	126	131	136	142	147	153	158	164	191	218
5'3"	107	113	118	124	130	135	141	146	152	158	163	169	197	225
5'4"	110	116	122	128	134	140	145	151	157	163	169	174	204	232
5'5"	114	120	126	132	138	144	150	156	162	168	174	180	210	240
5'6"	118	124	130	136	142	148	155	161	167	173	179	186	216	247
5'7"	121	127	134	140	146	153	159	166	172	178	185	191	223	255
5'8"	125	131	138	144	151	158	164	171	177	184	190	197	230	262
5'9"	128	135	142	149	155	162	169	176	182	189	196	203	236	270
5'10"	132	139	146	153	160	167	174	181	188	195	202	207	243	278
5'11"	136	143	150	157	165	172	179	186	193	200	208	215	250	286
6'0"	140	147	154	162	169	177	184	191	199	206	213	221	258	294
6'1"	144	151	159	166	174	182	189	197	204	212	219	227	265	302
6'2"	148	155	163	171	179	186	194	202	210	218	225	233	272	311
6'3"	152	160	168	176	184	192	200	208	216	224	232	240	279	319
6'4"	156	164	172	180	189	197	205	213	221	230	238	246	287	328

Each entry gives the body weight in pounds (lb.) for a person of a given height and body mass index. Pounds have been rounded off.

To use the table, find the appropriate height in the left-hand column. Move across the row to a given weight. The number at the top of the column is the body mass index for that height and weight.

Adapted from Bray, G.A., Gray, D.S. Obesity Part 1. Pathogenesis. West.J.Med. 1988, 149: 429-41

In January 2003, I compared the visceral body fat findings of 20 students to their body mass index. The data from the BMI indicated 15 students were at healthy weights, one student was overweight and four were obese. The visceral fat statistics were much different. Four students had optimal body fat. Seven had moderately high levels, three had high levels and six were very high. In Figure 4.2, Futrex Inc. has charted these numbers and separated them by gender.

FIGURE 4.2

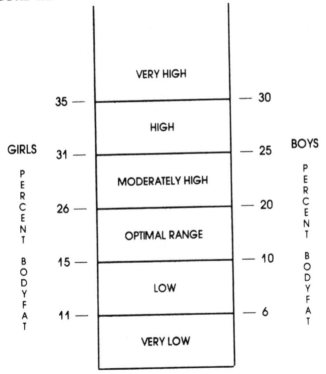

BODYFAT RECOMMENDATIONS AGES 5 THRU 17
CONFORMS TO AAHPERD 1989 FITNESS STANDARDS

Unfortunately, this means the unhealthy fat is not even being considered in all of the statistics of obese Americans and yet this is the most dangerous fat. For comparison, Figure 4.3, Futrex Inc. also has charted the visceral body fat index for adults.

FIGURE 4.3

BESTEST
MEDICAL

17853 Santiago Boulevard
Suite 107-504
Villa Park, CA 92861
800-638-8739
(FAX) 714-693-2923
www.Bestest.com

"RATING SCALE"

Many people desire a "rating system" for assessing their current level of body fat. The following table provides a meaningful rating system.

MALE
(MAXIMUM PERCENTAGE TO FALL WITHIN THE GUIDELINES)

	RISKY	EXCELLENT	GOOD	FAIR	POOR	VERY POOR
19-24	<6%	10.8%	14.9%	19.0%	23.3%	>23.3%
25-29		12.8%	16.5%	20.3%	24.4%	
30-34		14.5%	18.0%	21.5%	25.2%	
35-39		16.1%	19.4%	22.6%	26.1%	
40-44		17.5%	20.5%	23.6%	26.9%	
45-49		18.6%	21.5%	24.5%	27.6%	
50-54		19.8%	22.7%	25.6%	28.7%	
55-59		20.2%	23.2%	26.2%	29.3%	
60+		20.3%	23.5%	26.7%	29.8%	

FEMALE

	RISKY	EXCELLENT	GOOD	FAIR	POOR	VERY POOR
19-24	<11%	18.9%	22.1%	25.0%	29.6%	>29.6%
25-29		18.9%	22.4%	25.4%	29.8%	
30-34		19.7%	22.7%	26.4%	30.5%	
35-39		21.0%	24.0%	27.7%	31.5%	
40-44		22.6%	25.6%	29.3%	32.8%	
45-49		24.3%	27.3%	30.9%	34.1%	
50-54		26.6%	29.7%	33.1%	36.2%	
55-59		27.4%	30.7%	34.0%	37.3%	
60+		27.6%	31.0%	34.4%	38.0%	

The FUTREX 5000/XL, 5000AZL, and 5000AWL use data similar to the above tables. The actual data used in the instrument is provided for each year of age from 5 to 80. All percentages are compiled by the National Institutes of Health (NIH).

Another illustration of the importance of exercise comes from an adult patient. She was very fit and exercised regularly. Her visceral fat was at a healthy 22%. Then she went through some life changes and her exercises slacked. A year later her visceral fat was at 27%, a significant change. I diagnosed her with what I call jokingly "stalled cow disease."

Cows that are kept in stalls so they do not exercise and eat a diet high in refined carbohydrates and grains produce meat marbled with fat, which is more tender compared to the meat of free-roaming cattle or wild game. However, excess amounts of marbled fat are not desirable in humans.

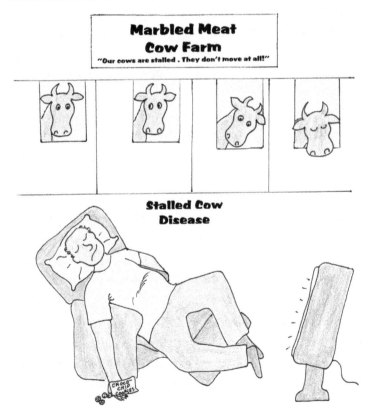

The benefits of regular cardiovascular exercise cannot be disputed. Recent research indicates the benefits may also include enhancing our memory. The hippocampus, a small organ inside the brain responsible for memory, shrinks with age. Regular cardiovascular exercise plumps it back up. Researchers now believe that memory loss and dementia may not be due to aging. They are caused by a sedentary lifestyle causing the hippocampus to shrink.

It is very important to understand the distinction between health and fitness. Health includes physical activity and some level of fitness. Fitness does not necessarily indicate health. I see cases in which persons lose weight, go to the gym and look fabulous. One or two years later they get very sick or experience catastrophic illnesses or death. People will say, "Why did that happen? I thought she or he was so healthy?"

First, I must point out, anything can happen to anyone at any time. Aside from that, weight loss due to calorie reduction and increased physical activity does not mean a person is getting quality calories. If the bulk of a person's diet is glue, plastic and refined sugars he or she can reduce weight by reducing calories, but good health requires quality calories.

Being overweight is often associated with poor health, but thinness does not guarantee good health. The way a person chooses to lose weight can be very hard on the body.

Athletes are another example of the difference between health and fitness. They may be fit, but many suffer devastating illnesses or untimely deaths from heart disease, stroke, cancer or other diseases. Athletes have been compared to the canary sent into the coal mine.

As the story goes, the canary would be sent into the coal mine and if it died, the humans stayed out. The canary was much more sensitive to the poison in air than a person would be. Because of the extra physical demands on an athlete's body, he or she has to work hard at being well nourished. Unfortunately, many of them don't take it seriously or they follow faulty advice leading them to eat non-nutritive products, consisting of refined grains, trans fats and refined sugars.

The experts are now stating that the upcoming generation will not outlive its parents because of current trends of child obesity, diabetes, heart disease and cancer. Most people wouldn't argue that our children are the nation's most valuable resource. They are not eating well. Young people are still developing the lifestyles that determine their pattern of choices concerning food and exercise. I am thrilled with the changes I see in a small group of students over a short period of time. With a minimum of teaching I've observed a significant change in understanding of food and measurable changes in behavior.

I feel we must get their attention and do something productive once we get it. The answer to my original question: "Do they know what is and is not healthy?" They do not. They need to be taught. We can't control what they will do with the information they are given, but from what I've seen with my students, more than we might expect. The first step is to just tell them.

One of the best stories Judy Powell shared with me was about a student who, after watching, listening and tasting my presentation, went home to excitedly share her new knowledge with her parents. The student pulled two chairs up to the family pantry so her parents could sit down. She proceeded to examine one item at a time, pointing out the partially hydrogenated fat, enriched wheat and high fructose corn syrup in each product.

She explained to her parents why these non-food substances had no place in their kitchen. This 14-year-old went home from school with a complete understanding of a new and very large concept that has the potential of altering her life. She was able to do this after only about three hours of classroom instruction and a trip to the grocery store.

I am saddened when I read the writings of experts who say that getting high school students to make any dietary changes is "virtually a waste of time." I disagree. It is my opinion that we must change our approach to teaching nutrition.

As long as they are getting the same generic and conflicting advice (reduce saturated fat and eat more vegetables, but don't put butter or salt on them, but drink more milk) they will continue to make detrimental choices. They study how to decipher the information listed in the nutrition facts box, but don't see why the choice for lower fat often means higher sugar. They don't understand that it really doesn't matter if the product has a few less grams of carbohydrates or fats. They are still eating glue and plastic.

The practical application of a nutrition class is for the students to eat better and be healthier, but it is lost in charts, percentages and long lists of words referring to isolated nutrients that are not whole foods. I think teens need a more tangible motivation to give up French fries and soda in favor of healthier meats, vegetables, and fruits. I taught them they were eating glue and plastic (literally), because that has an impact on them.

When I see their noses wrinkle, hear the gasps of shock and see the looks of disgust on their faces, I know they progressed at least one step forward. These non-nutritive products will not look the same to them.

* * * * * *

One final word on why we may want to choose better nourishment for our bodies. Most of us know of someone who is in his or her later years, seemingly ate all the wrong things, drank too much alcohol and probably smoked cigarettes. Against all odds they still appeared to thrive. They are not the norm. The picture is bigger than just one generation.

Many nutritional deficiencies reveal themselves in our children, grandchildren and great grandchildren. The infant mortality rate is a barometer of the health of a society. The United States doesn't rank well. Forty countries including Taiwan, Cuba and most European countries have lower infant mortality rates than the United States. We are one of the richest countries with the most advanced medical system and yet our babies are dying.

In studies done by Francis M. Pottenger, Jr. M.D., animals fed a nutritionally deficient diet for several generations reveal some shocking discoveries. By the third and fourth generations many of the offspring were sterile. Many had severe spinal and extremity malformations. They were unable to stand on four legs. Cancer, tumors, a multitude of diseases and birth defects appeared in the majority of the offspring of the third and fourth generations, which suffered from deficient nutrition.

When that same genetic line which had been bred with such nutritional deficiencies was fed a very nutrient dense diet, within three to fourth generations most of the diseases and birth defects were no longer present.

In 1871 after the fall of the Second Empire, the French government understood that to have a strong army of warriors they had to nourish the young women of child-bearing age. They knew it was important for the young women to be well nourished several months and even years before they conceived.

This insight was a new thought process for that time. In the surrounding regions the practice was to give the best food to the army so they could be stronger. The French government gave the most nutritious food to the future mothers. They knew this would produce the strongest army.

I teach about superior nutrition because I want to encourage people to feed themselves and their children as if Eternity was looking over their shoulders.

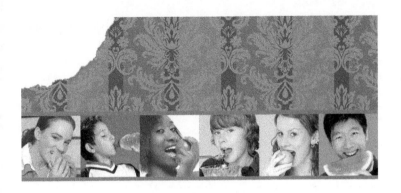

CHAPTER 5
Food Choices and Meal Planning

Now I will get practical and explain how to get you started on a healthier way to eat. Remember the chart (Fig. 1.1 on page 11) containing the regenerative and degenerative foods? We'll begin there.

Take a piece of paper and divide it into eleven columns. Label the columns with these words: vegetables, fruits, meat/eggs, dairy, beans/legumes, whole grains, herbs/seasonings, condiments/spreads/oils, nuts/seeds, sweeteners, beverages as seen in Figure 5.1 on the following page.

List your favorite foods in the appropriate columns, keeping in mind only regenerative foods. For me, a partial list for me might look like Figure 5.2, which you can view on page 76.

Post this paper with all these foods on your refrigerator. The next time you say, "What can I eat?" "What would be healthy?" You have a list in front of you. A meal is simply a combination of some of these foods.

FIGURE 5.1

VEGETABLES	FRUITS	MEAT/EGGS	DAIRY	BEANS/ LEGUMES (peas/lentils)
_____	_____	_____	_____	_____
_____	_____	_____	_____	_____
_____	_____	_____	_____	_____
_____	_____	_____	_____	_____
_____	_____	_____	_____	_____
_____	_____	_____	_____	_____
_____	_____	_____	_____	_____
_____	_____	_____	_____	_____
_____	_____	_____	_____	_____
_____	_____	_____	_____	_____
_____	_____	_____	_____	_____

WHOLE GRAINS	HERBS/ SEASONINGS	CONDIMENTS/ SPREADS/OILS	NUTS/ SEEDS
_____	_____	_____	_____
_____	_____	_____	_____
_____	_____	_____	_____
_____	_____	_____	_____
_____	_____	_____	_____
_____	_____	_____	_____
_____	_____	_____	_____
_____	_____	_____	_____
_____	_____	_____	_____
_____	_____	_____	_____
_____	_____	_____	_____

SWEETNERS	BEVERAGES
_____	_____
_____	_____
_____	_____
_____	_____
_____	_____
_____	_____
_____	_____
_____	_____
_____	_____
_____	_____

FIGURE 5.2

VEGETABLES	FRUITS	MEAT/EGGS	DAIRY
Broccoli	Apples	Orange Roughy	Cottage Cheese
Summer squash	Pears	Salmon	Cheddar Cheese
Potatoes	Strawberries	Cod	Feta Cheese
Tomatoes	Blueberries	Roast Beef	Romano Cheese
Mushrooms	Pineapple	Filet Mignon	Parmesan Cheese
Mixed greens	Lemons	Turkey	Swiss Cheese
Carrots	Raspberries	Mahi Mahi	Provolone Cheese
Cucumbers	Blackberries	Tuna	Cream Cheese
Garlic	Raisins	Ground Beef	Heavy Cream
Onions	Bananas	Pirch	Gorgonzola Cheese
Avocadoes	Oranges	Chicken	Bleu Cheese
Red/yellow peppers	Grapes	Shrimp	Asagio Cheese

BEANS/ LEGUMES	WHOLE GRAINS	HERBS/ SEASONINGS	CONDIMENTS/ SPREAD OILS
Edaname	Brown Rice	Basil	Olive Oil
Pinto Beans	Whole Wheat Pasta	Oregano	Butter
Red Beans	Brown Rice Pasta	Rosemary	Peanut Oil
Black Beans	Sprouted grain bread	Celtic Salt	Coconut oil
Garbanzo Beans	Spelt	Nutmeg	Hummus
Navy Beans	Sprouted grain pita-	Cinnamon	Toasted-
Lentils	bread	Cumin	Sesame oil
Split Peas	Cornmeal	Turmeric	Olives
Adzuki Beans	Steel cut oats	Dill	mustard
Kidney Beans	Barley	Mint	
Black-eyed peas	Wild rice	Curry	
Green Beans	Sprouted grain buns	Pepper	
	Quinoa		

NUTS/SEEDS	SWEETNERS	BEVERAGES
Sunflower Seeds	Honey	Water
Pecans	Maple Syrup	Green Tea
Walnuts	Raw Cane Sugar	Black Tea
Almonds	Brown Rice Syrup	Red Tea
Brazil Nuts	Succinate	White Tea
Peanuts	Rapadura Sugar	Homemade-
Peanut Butter	Molasses	Fruit Water
Pistachio nuts	Black Strap Molasses	Coffee
Pumpkin seeds	Tubinado sugar	Lemon water
Flax seeds		Twig tea
Hazel nuts		Mint tea
Cashews		

The following is an example of how I combine the foods I enjoy to make meals for three days:

Day one:

Breakfast

Eggs

Sprouted grain toast with butter

Lemon water

Lunch

Lentil soup

Apple with peanut butter

Lemon water

Dinner

Broiled cod (marinade in fresh squeezed lime juice and salt for 15 minutes and broil 10 minutes or less)

Steamed broccoli

Sprouted grain bread with olive oil and Romano cheese broiled for 2-3 minutes

Sliced tomatoes

Baby carrots

Sliced red peppers

I prepare a plate of raw vegetables every day for lunch or dinner if I don't prepare a salad. It is very quick and easy. I will add different cheeses and olives with a variety of three or four raw vegetables.

Day two:

Breakfast

Cottage cheese with fresh strawberries and raw walnuts

Slice of sprouted grain bread with butter

Lemon water

Lunch

Salad: mixed greens, cherry tomatoes, grated carrots, chopped yellow peppers, soybeans (edemame), raisins, sunflower seeds, feta cheese (no dressing)

Dinner

Boiled brown rice

Red beans

Peas

Plate of celery, cucumbers, sliced tomatoes, cheese, olives

Dessert: thinly sliced apple drizzled with honey and cinnamon

Lemon or fruit water* or green tea

*To make fruit water, fill a two-quart glass pitcher with filtered water and add any favorite fruit, 1/2 cup or more. Let set for four hours. My favorite is a mix of strawberries, blueberries, raspberries, blackberries and fresh pineapple with a little of its own juice. After four hours or overnight remove the fruit (it will be blanched) and discard.

Day three:

Breakfast

Egg omelet with red peppers, onions, green squash, cheddar cheese and mushrooms

Sprouted grain toast with butter

Lemon water

Lunch

Sandwich on sprouted grain bread (heated, not toasted), made with mayonnaise, tomatoes, avocado, cheese and lettuce

Sliced pears and cherries
Lemon water
Dinner
Grilled steak
Black beans
Steamed spinach
Sliced tomatoes
Fruit water

I realize I need to suggest snacks and desserts and they, too, can be healthy choices. Here are some ideas:

- Diced apple, raisins and pecans
- Strawberries and blueberries with whipped cream
- Nectarines with a handful of pistachio nuts
- Avocados and grapes
- Grapes and cheese
- Peanut butter (freshly ground) and apple
- Peanut butter with celery or carrots
- Banana split: slice a banana and place one or two scoops of cottage cheese between the slices; top with strawberries, blueberries and/or walnuts, etc.

I frequently make a fruit smoothie for my breakfast. I use whatever fruit I have on hand, which is usually what is in season. One example is to combine a banana, a nectarine, half of a cup of mixed berries: blueberries, raspberries, strawberries and blackberries with water in the blender.

I also add a Standard Process whole foods powder for additional superior nutrition. The powder includes ingredients such as whey protein, flax meal powder, brown rice protein powder, buckwheat juice powder, brussels sprouts (the whole plant), kale, barley grass, alfalfa juice powder, carrot powder and a few other ingredients, such as lecithin. The vegetables are dehydrated without heat in a vacuum. This means they still contain all their nutrients (thousands of them) including enzymes. This is an excellent alternative to popular sugar-laden protein powders.

These are just some examples of how you can take a list of favorite foods and combine them for meals and snacks. I did not include any baked desserts or so-called "healthy cookies," because they are not part of my daily staples. Remember, if we eat superior nutrition 90 percent of the time, most of us can eat up to ten percent of what I call "poison". My recommendation is to try to satisfy a sweet tooth with fruit and the craving for fats with nuts, cheese and meats. Also, I drink water with lemon throughout the day, not just with meals. Proper hydration helps in all areas of health from proper gastrointestinal functioning to anti-aging benefits.

* * * * * *

I hear many questions about hormones and antibiotics in meat and pesticides on fresh produce. If you can find and afford hormone and antibiotic free meat, it is a better choice. If you can buy organic or locally grown produce that is pesticide-free, then do. However, replacing meat that contains hormones or antibiotics or produce that has been treated with pesticides with glue, plastic and refined sugars is not a good choice.

The average person eats 25-30 different foods as his or her staples. The list of an average person might include doughnuts, hamburgers, French fries, chips, pretzels and other processed snacks.

We are taught that variety is good for us and gives us a wider array of nutrients. I agree. But for many, that can be overwhelming, so I start with simply listing foods you know and like, even if it is only 25-30. To begin a healthy eating pattern, go ahead and eat your favorites.

Most people experience what I call withdrawal symptoms when they go off the processed and refined foods. One of the complaints is that the food doesn't taste as good. Real food has its own taste, which is subtle compared to all the exaggerated flavors in processed and refined foods. The taste buds have to be allowed time to appreciate the taste of real food. When a person walks out of a rock concert, he or she can't hear birds singing. His or her ears have been over-stimulated. It is the same when you change from processed foods to real and whole foods. Your taste buds need time to detect the subtle flavors

Another complaint I hear is an increase in salt and sugar cravings, which have become even stronger. That is because you have given up things like soda and chips, which are very high in sugar and salt. I recommend using a healthier sea salt, such as Celtic Sea Salt or Redmond Sea Salt on meats, vegetables, beans and other foods. Just a little amount goes a long way to enhance the flavor.

As long as you are eating fresh food at home, your salt intake will be less than eating processed food, which is commonly very high in commercial grade salt. Some good quality salt is important in our diets. It helps regulate body temperature. A quality sea salt also adds over 60 trace minerals to our diets.

A third complaint I hear is some people miss the baked goods and more complex desserts. There are a multitude of cookbooks on the market that teach how to bake with whole grains and healthy sweeteners for baked goods and desserts. And, now that you are eating better, you may actually seek to change the way you bake.

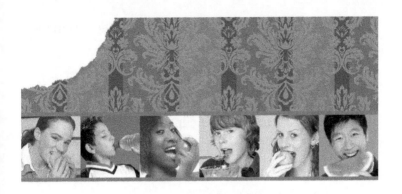

CHAPTER 6

Recipes to Get You Started

I want to illustrate how easy and fun eating good can be. Here are some of my favorite recipes.

SALMON QUICHE 》

My mother made this quiche while I was growing up.

For the crust:

>1 cup of whole wheat flour
>
>2/3 cup shredded sharp cheddar cheese
>
>1/2 teaspoon salt
>
>6 tablespoons olive oil
>
>1/4 cup slivered almonds
>
>1/4 teaspoon paprika
>
>*Combine all ingredients and press into a pie pan for the crust.*

Filling:

One 15-oz. can of wild salmon (reserve the liquid and add water to make 1/2 cup)

3 eggs, beaten

1 cup of sour cream

1/4 cup mayonnaise

1/2 cup shredded sharp cheddar cheese

1 tablespoon grated onion

1/4 teaspoon dried dill weed

3 to 5 shakes Tabasco Sauce

Remove the skin and bones from the salmon, flake the meat and set aside. Combine the eggs, sour cream and mayonnaise. Add the cheese, onion, dill and Tabasco Sauce. Add salmon and water. Mix and pour into the crust. Bake at 400 F° for 10 minutes. Reduce heat to 325 F° and continue baking for 45 minutes. Cool before serving.

ANNIE'S ZUCCHINI PIZZA CRUST ≫

Preheat oven to 350 F°

3-1/2 cups slightly salted grated zucchini

1/3 cup whole grain flour

1/2 cup parmesan cheese

3 eggs

1/2 cup mozzarella cheese

Pinch of spices of choice (i.e. basil, oregano)

> *Salt the zucchini lightly and let sit for 15 minutes, drain excess moisture. Combine zucchini with remaining ingredients and spread on oiled pan. Bake 20-25 minutes until dry. Brush with olive oil and broil for five minutes. Add favorite toppings and heat again for 25 minutes.*

This pizza crust recipe is from my friend, Annie, which is why I call it Annie's Pizza Crust. This is an excellent crust for diabetics. One of my friends, a diabetic, makes this almost every week. She won a prize for submitting it to a magazine and was filmed and interviewed by the magazine while making it.

I make my own pizza sauce. I start by heating olive oil in a saucepan. I add finely chopped fresh garlic, cook until you start to smell the garlic, then add finely chopped Vidalia onions. Let simmer briefly and add diced, fresh tomato, basil, oregano and salt. Cook on low for a few minutes before adding one 6 oz. can of tomato paste. Mix well and cook on low for about 30 minutes.

While sauce is cooking, cut up fresh vegetables and grate cheese. I use a variety of fresh vegetables and cheeses for toppings. These are examples of vegetables: spinach, mushrooms, red, orange, yellow and green peppers, black olives, green olives and broccoli. I use these cheeses: mozzarella, sharp cheddar, parmesan, romano, asagio and/or feta.

I have fun mixing various combinations together to create an endless variety of pizzas. When I invite friends over for pizza, I double or triple the crust and sauce recipes. It is also good left over.

LENTIL SOUP »

I like to make homemade soups. One of my favorite cookbooks is Aveline Kushi's Complete Guide to Macrobiotic Cooking. I often make alterations to suite my own tastes. This is my version of her lentil soup.

- 1 cup of dried lentils
- 2 sweet Vidalia onions, diced
- 1 carrot, diced
- 2 celery stalks, diced
- 1 quart of spring or filtered water
- 1/2 teaspoon sea salt (divided)
- 1 tablespoon Parsley, chopped

Wash the lentils and drain. Layer vegetables in a pot, starting with the onions, followed by the carrots and celery. Spread the lentils on top. Add water and a pinch of salt. Bring to a boil. Reduce heat to low, cover and simmer for 45 minutes. Add the chopped parsley and remaining salt. Simmer for 20 minute longer. Serve.

Layering the vegetables enhances the flavors so don't stir the soup while it is cooking. If you use different vegetables, remember to place the more dense ones in the bottom and work your way up.

CORN BREAD »

I like to have fresh bread with homemade soup. I particularly enjoy corn bread. This recipe comes from the

Arrowhead Mills package of organic yellow cornmeal. I have made a few minor changes for my personal preference.

> 1-1/2 cups Arrowhead Mills yellow cornmeal
>
> 1/2 cup spelt four
>
> 4 teaspoons aluminum-free baking powder (Rumford Baking Powder qualifies)
>
> 1/2 teaspoon sea salt
>
> 1cup cream
>
> 1 egg
>
> 1/2 cup water
>
> 2 tablespoons non-refined sugar

In a large bowl, combine all dry ingredients. Add all liquid ingredients. Mix well. Pour into a no. 8 well-oiled cast iron skillet and bake at 425 F° for 15-20 minutes. Eat while hot with honey and butter.

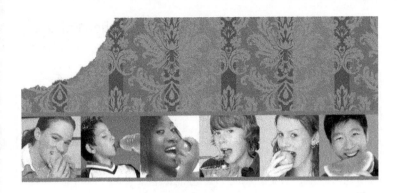

CHAPTER 7
Excerpts from Letters Written by Students

Judy Powell, the director of the health academy, asked her students to write a short note to me expressing their thoughts about my program. I thought they were all very encouraging. I have chosen two letters to include in their entirety. I will also share some excerpts of several others.

Dear Dr. Nancy,

You surprised me. I thought when Mrs. Powell told us that we were going to be learning about nutrition, that we'd be learning something pretty boring. Not something life changing! I can't tell you how much this helped my family and I eat better.

After going home and telling my dad that we shouldn't be eating this food, he didn't believe me – *at first*. Then after he found out that his sugar was becoming high and that he needed to watch what he ate...well, that's when he began to listen. I learned so much about the foods we eat and how half of the ones I loved were *so* unhealthy. I remember going through all of our foods and placing the ones that were horrible for us to eat on the counter, then pointing out what you explained to us. Even though everybody groaned, hating to throw away these 'good' tasting foods, we did. We did it to make the change and become healthy Americans...unlike most.

Now, we shop for healthy foods. Plenty of the ones you pointed out and small meals at home that we can make out of healthy foods. Lately, I've been feeling positive about everything and more energized. When my uncle came over to see our family, he brought over McDonalds...and I'll tell you one thing, a couple of those fries made me feel as if I was going to throw up. *You were completely right.* I got so used to healthy food, that when I look at this greasy, average day food us Americans eat, I felt sick.

I'm so very glad that you spent your time to teach my class and me about all these nasty foods we are eating on a daily basis. But, you didn't leave it there. You taught us even more – by explaining all the healthy foods we could eat and how much they helped. I thank you so very much, Dr. Nancy. I know if you weren't there, teaching us about these foods, I probably would be stuck eating very unhealthy foods. Thank you, once again, for taking time out of your schedule to come and see us.

Sincerely,

Jessica Sanchez

Dear Dr. Nancy

What is a *Hero*? Most people don't know the answer to this question or when they hear it they think of the comic book superheroes like Spiderman or Superman. A hero could be a police officer, a firefighter, a doctor, or pretty much anyone who helps save lives. Since the minute I was born I was eating bad foods. I was on a one way ticket to obesity, heart problems, diabetes, and maybe even death. It wasn't until fifteen years later that I realized my mistakes. It took a nutritionist named Nancy Irven to show me and my fellow classmates what we were doing wrong. After your first visit I understood what I was doing wrong.

First I had to cut out my white breads and replace them with 100% Whole Wheat bread and Ezekiel bread. At first I wasn't too psyched out about the whole idea because I thought that it would be dry and nasty but after having some with bananas, peanut butter, and honey I discovered a new joy. Ever since then everything that I eat that involves bread I have my Ezekiel right there next to me.

After that I had to work on the amount of plastic I was consuming. This was the hardest task to complete, mainly because every label that I read had the words "partially hydrogenated" in it. I found it everywhere while I was shopping in the stores mostly on cake mixes and the so called "Lean Gourmet" micro meals. So after seeing all that junk I made sure that I stayed away from that horrible stuff. Now I have been eating a lot of proteins. My favorite meal is my homemade healthy chicken salad sandwich on Ezekiel bread. I don't know what I would do without it.

The next killer was the addicting "high fructose corn syrup". I found this in a lot of things that I loved such as Gatorade, Ketchup, certain salad dressings, and my absolute favorite barbeque sauce. After seeing that on the labels I was thinking "know wonder I love all these foods." It was another challenge that I eventually came over.

If I were to have kept on going with my life eating all these bad foods around me then I guarantee you that I would have ended up with either heart problems or diabetes or death at an early age. Now let me ask the question again, "What is a *Hero*?" A hero is sometimes unknown as a hero. They are not seen as a hero, but Dr. Nancy when I look at you I see a <u>Hero</u>. It takes a special person to help save other people. You knew that one day we would all be in trouble with our health because of our eating habits. So you took the time and the money and the effort to show us and the past classes before us how we can prevent our mistakes by taking affirmative actions early. Just think of all the kids' lives you are saving, I know personally that <u>you have helped save my future life</u>. You are a hero in my heart and <u>I Thank You</u>.

Love always,

Anthony R. Bower

Anthony R. Bower

Dear Dr. Nancy,

" ...I have been reading lots of labels and have been making my own fresh fruit smoothies. Before you came to speak to us, I never ate breakfast and I ate tons of trans fat. I feel so healthy now. And I have lots of energy..."

* * * * * *

"I really liked the shakes. They were very good. I showed my mom how to make them; she really liked it just as much as I did. I believe I have been eating better. I have been trying to eat at least one raw food a day. I feel even better than before..."

* * * * * *

"You may have saved a couple of our lives from teaching us the right foods to eat so some day we don't end up with poor nutrition related health problems for example, heart attack, diabetes or stroke ... Please continue to educate people in the future on good nutrition and help to maybe save their lives, too."

* * * * * *

"Who knew that you could make healthy snacks that are made in minutes and that cost next to nothing? I also found myself not very hungry the rest of the day, which is very good for me because I always find myself eating and grabbing another snack.

Thanks to you I may be adding a few years onto my life by eating healthier and taking care of myself."

* * * * * *

"As a matter of fact, you have shown me how to eat healthy and still eat the things I like. I'm slowly beginning to shift my diet, because I know that my eating habits will affect me in the future ... You were right, eating healthy does make a person feel better."

* * * * * *

"I ... learned that most so called 'healthy foods' are really not too great after all. Thanks to you, I now know how to make easy, inexpensive and, most of all, healthy meals. I found myself not hungry for the rest of the day because the health food fills me up much better, as I have learned."

* * * * * *

"Before you came I barely knew anything about healthy foods and what to look for in the ingredient labels. Everyday after you came into our class I would go home and tell my mother all about what I had learned."

* * * * * *

"Before you came I was unaware of things like hydro-genated oils, enriched flour and high fructose corn syrup. I have recently started checking all my food labels and have been very astonished at what I have come across. Since you began your program I have made many changes in my eating lifestyle."

* * * * * *

"I'm here to thank you for taking your time to come to our Health Academy class and explain to us the nutritional facts that we probably never would have learned if it had not been for you ... Learning to read labels is another very interesting technique that you taught us. It has literally haunted me ever since you taught us that. I won't take a sip or bite of anything without first examining the label. Cookies, chips and soda were a big deal at my house before. Yeah, we knew they were bad, but they were just too good to resist. Now that we know what's really in them and what they do to our bodies, I haven't seen them in our house for a while. I mean, who would, if they knew that they were made out of glue and plastic."

* * * * * *

"I don't think, since you've come to see us, that I've looked at any food the same way. I'm constantly looking for bad ingredients and have turned to more nutritious snacks, such as fruit and vegetables instead of chips and candy. The list you had us write out with all the different food groups and what we liked in them is still up on my 'fridge and goes with my mother and I every time we go to the grocery store. I was amazed at how many different foods there really were that were so much better than the junk that everyone has grown to think was healthy."

* * * * * *

"Thank you for all the time and knowledge you shared with my class and me. Before you came I thought Powerade, white bread, pretzels and margarine were good for me. I also didn't have a clue about trans fat or refined grains. Of course, I have been lectured about it, but it was a boring subject to me and it just wasn't explained in an interesting way that I easily understood. I thank you for lecturing to me in a fun way. It was funny how you compared them to glue and plastic (this also served as an eye opener to many, not just me). Now I use butter, eat fruit for breakfast and avoid pretzels and Powerade. I also no longer eat plain white bread for a snack..."

* *

This book is not meant to be a complete prescription for all the areas of lifestyle change necessary for optimal health. I wanted to present a very simple plan to help my readers start eating more nutritious food, while still enjoying food. My years of experience have taught me that adults and young people are very confused about what is healthy and what is not. Knowing which healthy foods you like and learning to make them diet staples is the very beginning of better health.

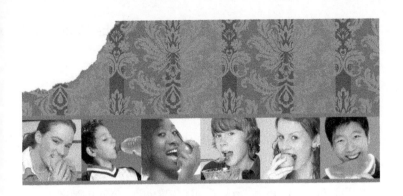

REFERENCES

Agatston, MD., Arthur. *The South Beach Diet.* Rodale, Inc., 2003

Bannard, MD. *Food for Life.* New York: Crown Publishers, 1993.

Beard-Miller, PhD, Jennie; Stephen Colagiuri, MD, Thomas Wolever, PhD, MD,MS, and Kaye Foster-Panell. *The Glucose Revolution.* New York; Marlowe & Company, 1999.

Brownstein, M.D., David. *Salt Your Way to Health.* West Bloomfield, MI: Medical Books Press, 2006.

Carmichael, Mary. "Stronger, Faster, Smarter." *Newsweek Magazine.* March 26, 2007.

Cataldo, Corinne Balog, Sharon Rady Rolfes, Eleanor Noss Whitney. *Understanding Clinical Nutrition.* Paul, MN: West Publishing Co., 1991.

Cordain, Ph.D., Loren. *The Paleo Diet*, Hoboken, NJ: John Wiley & Sons, Inc., 2002.

Davis, Adelle. *Let's Have Healthy Children*. New York: Harcourt Brace Jovanovich, Inc., 1981.

Davis, Adelle. *Let's Cook It Right*. New York: Harcourt Brace Jovanovich, Inc., 1970.

D'Adamo, Peter J., MD. *Eat Right for Your Type*. New York: G. P. Putnam's Sons, 1996.

DePuydt, Rita. *Baking With Stevia*. Oak View, CA: Sun Coast Enterprises, 1997.

Diamond, Harvey and Marilyn. *Fit for Life*. New York: Warner Books, Inc., 1985.

Dufty, William. *Sugar Blues*. New York: Warner Books, Inc., 1975.

Fallon, Sally with Mary G. Enig, Ph.D. *Nourishing Traditions*. Washington: New Trends Publishing, Inc., 2001.

Frost, Mary, MA. *Going Back to the Basics of Human Health. Avoiding the Fads, the Trends and the Bold-Faced Lies*. United States of America: Mary Frost, 1997.

Gadsby, Susan. "The Nutrition Paradox." *Discover Magazine*, October, 2004.

Green, Lawrence W. *Community Health*. St. Louis: Times Mirror/Mosby College Publishing, 1990.

Harvard Women's Health Watch. "Dietary calcium may be better for bones than calcium pills." September, 2007, Vol 15, no. 1.

Harvard Women's Health Watch. "Abdominal Fat and What To Do About It." December, 2006, Vol 14, no. 4.

Harvard Women's Health Watch. "The Trouble With Trans Fat." March, 2004, Vol 11, no. 7.

Harvard Women's Health Watch. "Go With the Grain, the Whole Grain." December, 2003, Vol 11, no.4.

Heller, MS, RD, Samantha. "The Hidden Killer," *Men's Health*, September, 2003.

Jensen, Bernard and Mark Anderson. *Empty Harvest*. United States of America: Bernard Jensen, 1990.

Kushi, Aveline with Alex Jack. *Complete Guide to Macrobiotic Cooking*. New York: Warner Books, Inc., 1985.

Mason, Michael. "78: Dietary Study Jolts Scientists." *Discover Magazine*. January, 2005.

McDougall, Christopher. "The Greatest Medical Revolution of the Century Is About to Begin." *Men's Health*, December, 2005.

Miller, Saul and JoAnn Miller. *Food for Thought*. Englewood Cliffs, New Jersey: Prentice-Hall, Inc., 1979.

Ornish, MD, Dean. *Dr. Ornish's Program for Reversing Heart Disease*. New York: Ballantine Books, a division of Random House, Inc., 1996.

Pereira, Mark, "Blood, Sweat and Tears," Children's Hospital, Boston.

Pottenger, Jr., MD, Francis M. *Pottenger's Cats: A Study in Nutrition*. Lemon Grove, Ca: Price-Pottenger Nutrition Foundation, Inc., 1995. www.ppnf.org. 1800-366-3748.

Robbins, John. *Diet for a New America*. Walpole, NH: Stillpoint Publishing, 1987.

Sears, PhD, Barry. *A Week in the Zone*. New York: HarperCollins Publishers, Inc., 2000.

Shell, Ellen Ruppel. "Interior Designs." *Discover Magazine*. December 2004.

Simontacchi, Carol. *Crazy Makers, How the Food Industry Is Destroying Our Brains and Harming Our Children*. New York: Jeremy Tarcher/Putnam, a member of Penguin Putnam, Inc., 2000.

"Sweet Nothings," *Self Healing*. October 2003.

Vigilante, MD, MPH, Kevin and Mary Flynn, PhD. *Low Fat Lies*. Washington, DC: Life Line Press, 1999.

Willett, MD, Walter C. *Eat, Drink and Be Healthy*. The Harvard Medical School Guide to Healthy Eating. New York: Simon & Schuster, 2003.

Williams, Sue Rodwell. *Nutrition and Diet Therapy, 6th Edition*. St. Louis: Times Mirror/Mosby College Publishing, 1989.

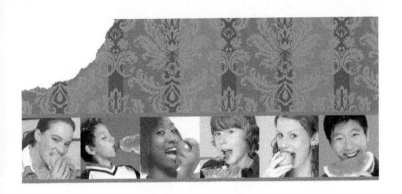

SUGGESTED READING

Ettlinger, Steve Twinkie, *Deconstructed*. New York: Penguin Press, 2007.

Gratzer, Walter. *Terror of the Table*. New York: Oxford University Press, 2005.

Jensen, Bernard and Mark Anderson. *Empty Harvest*. United States of America, Bernard Jensen, 1990.

Pollan, Michael. *Omnivore's Dilemma*. New York: Penguin Press, 2006.

Simontacchi, Carol. *Crazy Makers, How the Food Industry Is Destroying Our Brains and Harming Our Children*. New York: Jeremy Tarcher/Putnum, a member of Penguin Putnam, Inc., 2000.

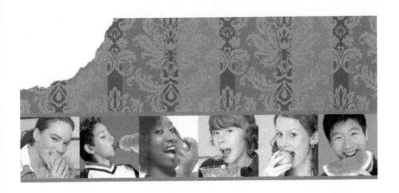

ABOUT THE AUTHOR

Nancy Inskeep Irven, D.C., is a practicing chiropractor in Crystal River, Florida. She has been in practice since 1994.

In 1999 she earned her Health Practitioner Diplomate in the clinical sciences of anti-aging medicine from the American Board of Anti-Aging Health Practitioners.

Dr. Irven has designed a unique program to assess the nutritional needs of patients. Her recommendations are based on the biochemical individuality of each one. She also assesses their visceral body fat, several biomarkers, and a blood profile of at least thirty-four tests

She lives in Crystal River, Florida, with her husband, Carl, himself a retired chiropractor.

ABOUT THE ILLUSTRATOR »

Paulette Lash Ritchie is a freelance journalist. She is the editor of a local magazine. She has been a newspaper reporter for 13 years and has had stories and/or art in several periodicals. She has been drawing since childhood.

Mrs. Ritchie lives in Floral City, Florida with her husband, Tom, and two children, Laura Lee and Luke, who are all learning better eating habits.